AF333625

DILEMMAS IN DIABETES

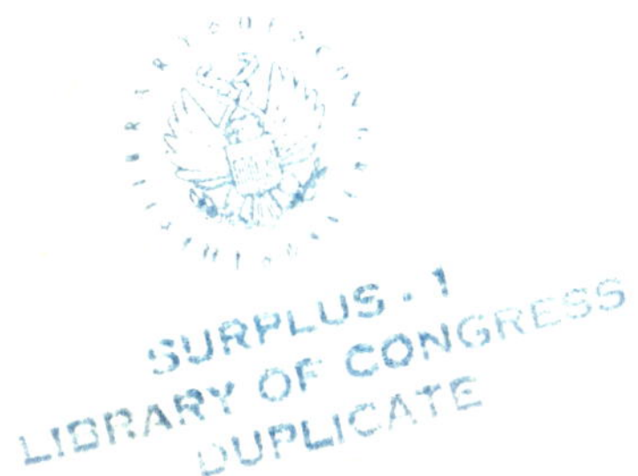
SURPLUS - 1
LIBRARY OF CONGRESS
DUPLICATE

ADVANCES IN EXPERIMENTAL MEDICINE AND BIOLOGY

Editorial Board:

Nathan Back   *State University of New York at Buffalo*

N. R. Di Luzio   *Tulane University School of Medicine*

Bernard Halpern   *Collège de France and Institute of Immuno-Biology*

Ephraim Katchalski   *The Weizmann Institute of Science*

David Kritchevsky   *Wistar Institute*

Abel Lajtha   *New York State Research Institute for Neurochemistry and Drug Addiction*

Rodolfo Paoletti   *University of Milan*

Recent Volumes in this Series

Volume 55
CONCANAVALIN A
Edited by Tushar K. Chowdhury and A. Kurt Weiss • 1975

Volume 56
BIOCHEMICAL PHARMACOLOGY OF ETHANOL
Edited by Edward Majchrowicz • 1975

Volume 57
THE SMOOTH MUSCLE OF THE ARTERY
Edited by Stewart Wolf and Nicholas T. Werthessen • 1975

Volume 58
CYTOCHROMES P-450 and b_5: Structure, Function, and Interaction
Edited by David Y. Cooper, Otto Rosenthal, Robert Snyder,
and Charlotte Witmer • 1975

Volume 59
ALCOHOL INTOXICATION AND WITHDRAWAL: Experimental Studies II
Edited by Milton M. Gross • 1975

Volume 60
DIET AND ATHEROSCLEROSIS
Edited by Cesare Sirtori, Giorgio Ricci, and Sergio Gorini • 1975

Volume 61
EXPLORATIONS IN AGING
Edited by Vincent J. Cristofalo, Jay Roberts, and Richard C.
Adelman • 1975

Volume 62
CONTROL MECHANISMS IN DEVELOPMENT: Activation, Differentiation,
and Modulation in Biological Systems
Edited by Russel H. Meints and Eric Davies • 1975

Volume 63
LIPIDS, LIPOPROTEINS, AND DRUGS
Edited by David Kritchevsky, Rodolfo Paoletti, and
William L. Holmes • 1975

Volume 64
IMMUNOLOGIC PHYLOGENY
Edited by W. H. Hildemann and A. A. Benedict • 1975

Volume 65
DILEMMAS IN DIABETES
Edited by Stewart Wolf and Beatrice Bishop Berle • 1975

Totts Gap Colloquium on Diabetes Mellitus, Totts Gap, Penn, 1974.

DILEMMAS IN DIABETES

Edited by

Stewart Wolf

The Marine Biomedical Institute
The University of Texas Medical Branch at Galveston

and

Beatrice Bishop Berle

Albert Einstein College of Medicine

PLENUM PRESS • NEW YORK AND LONDON

RC
660
T722
1974

Library of Congress Cataloging in Publication Data

Totts Gap Colloquium on Diabetes Mellitus, 1974.
  Dilemmas in diabetes.

  (Advances in experimental medicine and biology; v. 65)
  Bibliography: p.
  Includes index.
  1. Diabetes—Congresses. I. Wolf, Stewart George, 1914-   II. Berle, Beatrice
Bishop, 1902   III. Title. IV. Series.
  RC660.A1T67 1974   616.4'62   75-33729
  ISBN 0-306-39065-5

Proceedings of the Totts Gap Colloquium on Diabetes Mellitus,
held in Totts Gap, Pennsylvania, May 9-11, 1974

Officers and Directors

John G. Bruhn, Ph.D., *President and Director*
Beatrice B. Berle, M.D., *Vice-President and Director*
Stewart Wolf, M.D., *Secretary Treasurer and Director*
Mr. George Plush, *Director*

Board of Trustees

Mark D. Altschule, M.D.   Robert C. Page, M.D.
William B. Bean, M.D.   Edmund D. Pellegrino, M.D.
Andre Cournand, M.D.   Eliot Stellar, Ph. D.
William C. Gibson, M.D.   Mr. Oscar Swarth
Miss Helen Goodell   Joseph M. White, M.D.
Franz J. Ingelfinger, M.D.

Advisory Council to Totts Gap Colloquia:

Mark D. Altschule, M.D.   Franz J. Ingelfinger, M.D.
Andre Cournand, M.D.   Mr. Oscar Swarth
Martin M. Cummings, M.D.   N. T. Werthessen, Ph.D.

© 1975 Plenum Press, New York
A Division of Plenum Publishing Corporation
227 West 17th Street, New York, N.Y. 10011

United Kingdom edition published by Plenum Press, London
A Division of Plenum Publishing Company, Ltd.
Davis House (4th Floor), 8 Scrubs Lane, Harlesden, London, NW10 6SE, England

All rights reserved

No part of this book may be reproduced, stored in a retrieval system, or transmitted,
in any form or by any means, electronic, mechanical, photocopying, microfilming,
recording, or otherwise, without written permission from the Publisher

Printed in the United States of America

This volume is dedicated to the memory of

I. Arthur Mirsky

who died at the age of 67, several weeks after the Colloquium in which he was to have participated. Dr. Mirsky, a physician, scientist, and scholar of rare quality, contributed richly to our present-day understanding of diabetes. His remarkable capacity for synthesis sprang from a mind both quick and judicious. His personal warmth, his fairness and dogged pursuit of truth endeared him to all who knew him well.

Preface

This volume contains the edited proceedings of the Totts Gap
Colloquium on Diabetes Mellitus, DILEMMAS IN DIABETES. The Colloquium, lasting two and a half days, was organized mainly as a dialogue among experts in the field with different disciplinary back-
grounds and, to some extent, differing points of view. The effort
was to synthesize existing knowledge, reconciling disparate data and
interpretation, and pointing up important areas of ignorance. Thus,
the book should serve not only as a summary of recent information
on diabetes, but as a reliable guide to the practicing physician as
he wades through often conflicting etiologic dogmas and therapeutic
practices.

The Colloquium was made possible through the generous support
of the Geigy Pharmaceutical Company and the conscientious and expert
coordination of Mr. Oscar Swarth.

The participants were:

> Dr. George F. Cahill, Boston, Massachusetts
> Dr. Harvey C. Knowles, Cincinnati, Ohio
> Dr. Rachmiel Levine, Duarte, California
> Dr. Lelio Orci, Geneva, Switzerland
> Dr. Norton Spritz, New York, New York
> Dr. Roger Unger, Dallas, Texas
> Dr. Robert Williams, Seattle, Washington
> Dr. Stewart Wolf, Galveston, Texas

Dr. Arnold Lazarow and Dr. I. Arthur Mirsky were to have participated, but unfortunately were ill at the time of the meeting.

Others in attendance included five medical students, especially
selected from medical schools in the Philadelphia/New York area.
They were:

> Mr. Louis Green, Univ. of Pennsylvania School of Medicine
> Dr. Steven Peiken, Jefferson Medical College

Dr. Alan Ropper, Cornell Univ. Medical College
Dr. Allan Schwartz, Columbia Univ. School of Medicine
Dr. Charles Rost, Temple Univ. School of Medicine

Four members of the Board of Trustees of the Totts Gap Institute
(Dr. Beatrice B. Berle, Miss Helen Goodell, Dr. Robert C. Page, and
Mr. Oscar Swarth) were present, as well as Miss Barbara Ramm and
Mr. Jerome Mattox from the Geigy Pharmaceutical Company.

Illustrations from the following publications have been reproduced with permission:

Diabetes
Journal of Clinical Investigation
Metabolism
New England Journal of Medicine

The editors acknowledge the devoted help of Mrs. Joan Martin,
assisted by Miss Colleen Hogan and Mrs. Cindy Carter.

Contents

Introduction

"More things are shewed unto thee than men understand."
                              - Eccliasticus 3: 23

Knowledge of the diabetic state and the metabolic aberrations associated with it has increased rapidly in the recent past. The pieces of the puzzle have become so numerous, however, that to put them together into a coherent picture has become more difficult instead of less so. Instead of affording a clearer rationale for therapy, the vast accumulation of information has brought into question some of our most cherished therapeutic dogmas.

The concept of pre-diabetes, once widely accepted, is now seriously challenged. No longer is lability of blood sugar regulation a reliable harbinger of clinical diabetes mellitus. Capillary basement membrane thickening, once confidently attributed to sustained hyperglycemia has been found at times to precede the hyperglycemic state by several years. The role of growth hormone and the place of hypophysectomy in management are less certain than they once were.

The value of oral hypoglycemic therapy and even the actions of insulin are being examined. A variety of vexing problems concerning our understanding of diabetes has accumulated since the seeming finality of the therapeutic preparation of insulin in 1927. Therefore, in an effort to synthesize available knowledge and to reconcile disparate data and interpretation, leading experts in the field were brought together for informal dialogue.

Chapter I - HISTORICAL PERSPECTIVE

     DR. LEVINE: Before actually tackling the dilemma of the relat-
ionship of pancreatic function to diabetes mellitus, I should point
out that early etiologic concepts did not even take the pancreas into consideration.

     Following the discovery by Thomas Willis that diabetic urine
was sweet (147) and after Dobson evaporated diabetic urine and saw
"candy" as a residue, (29) the natural inference was to implicate
a kidney disorder as the cause of diabetes. Cantharides, a kidney
poison, was therefore proposed as treatment. Perhaps the chronic
inflammation and scarring of glomeruli that resulted may have les-
sened glycosuria, but surely it did not promote health or longevity.
Years later Rollo discovered the influence of diet on the degree of
severity of glycosuria (118). Observing the different effects of
carbohydrates, of proteins and of fats, he implicated the stomach
and gastro-intestinal tract as the primary organs affected in diabetes. Despite his erroneous inference, Rollo must be credited with
taking the first practical steps toward the modern dietary treatment
of diabetes. About the same time as Rollo (in 1776), Cawley published the results of an autopsy of a patient who died with diabetes
(19). He found that the pancreas was shriveled and full of calculi.
No contemporary paid any attention to this first mention of the pancreas as possibly implicated in diabetes. The physiologist, Conrad
Bruner in Switzerland, came close to making the discovery Minkowski
made 150 years later (15). He did pancreatectomies in dogs, and
noted that they urinated very frequently, but he did not examine
their urine.

     In the period from 1800 to 1889, the pancreatic lesions of
diabetes were rediscovered but their
The Pancreas as the   inconsistent presence led to contro-
Source of Diabetes   versy as to whether diabetes had a pan-
                           creatic etiology or not. Bouchardat,
Professor of Hygiene (Public Health) in the School of Public Health
at Paris, from the 1830's to the 1870's had an excellent background
in chemistry, imbibed from the French organic chemist, Chevreuil,
who was the first to determine that the sugar in diabetic urine is
glucose and differed from table sugar. He found at autopsy, damage
to the pancreas in 14 out of 19 wasted young people with heavy
glycosuria. On the basis of his findings, he divided diabetes into three etiological groups: Diabète Maigre (lean diabetes) which
he considered to be due to a pancreatic disturbance; Diabète Gras
(fat diabetes) in which the pancreas (he said) was not involved;
and a third group, Diabète Nerveuse. The latter he modelled on
Claude Bernard's "Piqure" of the floor of the fourth ventricle,
which is followed by glycosuria (11).

Actual production of the diabetic state by removal of the pancreas occurred in 1889. The islets of Langerhans had not yet been clearly identified, but the presence of non-acinar cell clusters in the pancreas was confirmed by Laguesse (72). At this point controversy was put aside and everyone accepted the pancreatic etiology of diabetes despite the fact that they could not find consistent characteristic lesions in man. Nevertheless, a text-book on diabetes published in 1898 by Naunyn, Minkowski's chief in Strasbourg (91) held to the multiple etiology for diabetes, giving at the same time enormous weight to the pancreatic form elucidated in his laboratory. A substance called "insulin" was postulated, and later in 1921, when Banting and Best showed that extracts of pancreas could lower blood sugar in all forms of diabetes, the pancreatic etiology seemed surely to have been established. A new uncertainty soon appeared, however, from Argentina, where Bernardo Houssay had demonstrated the amelioration of diabetic hyperglycemia by removal of the

Diabetogenic Effects of
Pituitary, Thyroid,
Adrenal and Liver

pituitary (59). His work was sparked by a review of Borchardt's in 1908, of a fairly recently described disease, Acromegaly (16). It inspired Houssay's experiments, which showed that experimental pancreatic diabetes in dogs could be modified to any desirable degree by a combination of diet and hypophysectomy. It is not generally appreciated that the degree of hyperglycemia following hypophysectomy will be directly related to the amount of carbohydrate and protein in the food. If there is no actual or potential carbohydrate in the food, the blood sugar will go down to a low level and even to zero; the more the animal will eat, the higher the hyperglycemia will be. Under all these circumstances there is little, if any, ketosis. Later it was shown that removal of the adrenals in the pancreatectomized animal gives a very similar picture to that of hypophysectomy. Finally, it was resolved that several factors in the pituitary were involved. One was ACTH, working by way of the adrenals; the other one was TSH (to some small extent) working via the thyroid; and the third, growth hormone, acting by, as yet, unknown ways. GH is an anti-insulin diabetogenic factor either directly or indirectly. All of this new knowledge, the work of Houssay, of Evans, of Young, and of Long and Lukens, as well as others finally led to a more modern version of the old multiple etiology of diabetes. The liver was considered the central organ, since the liver is essential to the production of hyperglycemia. After removal of the liver, the blood sugar falls to zero. A multitude of factors were known to play upon the liver — ACTH, thyroid, TSH, the growth hormone and adrenalin. All appeared as possible diabetogenic factors. Insulin was the only factor that counteracted these effects. Diabetes, therefore, was the result of an interplay between these factors, assuming the liver to be in a normal functional state. The liver itself could play a diabetogenic role because when it was disturbed in some way, glucose tolerance was also affected; for example, in hepatitis (early) or in cirrhosis (late) (127).

This understanding seemed to satisfy everyone fairly well up to the early 1940s when investigators began to measure the actual levels of hormones in the blood and tissues. Evidence of excess steroids, thyroid, or growth hormone, adrenalin, and so on, in diabetes were occasionally reported from various parts of the world, but most workers concluded that this multiple etiology, while theoretically true, could only concern a very, very small percentage of diabetics in the population. There were a few cases of acromegaly; there were a few cases of Cushing's disease; there were a few instances of hyperthyroidism with associated diabetes and even fewer of pheochromocytoma. It could be deduced that 99.9% of diabetics did not bear clinical or chemical stigmata of an excess of anti-insulin hormones. There was also very little evidence for hepatic etiology in any sizable group of diabetics. It appeared that the explanation would have to come from insulin lack rather than from excess of these other elements. However when insulin measurements became available they led to confusion. Blood insulin (in the juvenile form) was found to be very low, but the insulin in the adult-onset diabetes was not significantly different from that of the normal population of the same age, weight, sex, etc. The question, therefore, was and still is: if a single insulin-lack etiology is not proven for the vast majority of diabetics, if the hepatic etiology does not apply to any sizable number, and if the majority of people called diabetics have fasting insulins which approach the normal level, what has the pancreas to do with the disease? The next step was to refine the technique of insulin assay and then do the determinations frequently, not just a fasting value, but fasting as well as samples after stimulation of secretion by either a normal food intake or by the injection of glucose, aminoacids or other chemicals. At the present time, I think it is fair to say that most people will agree that a juvenile diabetic has a fasting insulin level which may or may not be lower than normal.

The Contrast of Juvenile and Adult Onset Diabetes

After stimulation, however, in a juvenile diabetic there is practically no change in the insulin level.

The puzzling finding was that in the adult-onset, non-ketotic diabetic, there is generally a higher than normal fasting insulin level. The degree of elevation is associated with the increased weight of these individuals. Obese non-diabetics also have a higher than normal fasting level that rises further with either a food or glucose stimulus. The rise is variable. Many feel that in diabetes there is a sluggish response of insulin secretion to a glucose load even though the fasting insulin level may be normal or high. The delay in insulin secretion and a decrease in the height or peak of insulin level following glucose, is interpreted by many to indicate that most diabetics have a deficient or faulty beta cell.

Luft and his group have pointed out (20) that the sluggish beta cell may constitute the characteristic of the genetic aspect

of diabetes, because it is also found in individuals who are genetically thought to be destined to have diabetes, so-called pre-diabetics
but who, at the time of these measurements, still had a perfectly normal glucose tolerance. Thus, Luft and his followers visualize a beta
cell which has lost its fine trigger-like response; something is wrong
with the gluco-receptor or transducer of the beta cell which makes it
sluggish. One must pause at this moment to point out that this is not
accepted by everybody. For example, workers in this country and
abroad have pointed out that not all new diabetics may have that kind
of delay at all (38). They may have a perfectly normal insulin
curve. Even though the peak may not be as high, the take-off and the
briskness of response was good. Therefore, there is no consensus of
opinion that all diabetes is <u>necessarily</u> insulin deficiency.

However, nothing has been substituted for the pancreas as an
etiological factor. In addition, one has
to stress the fact that the pancreas is
not just the seat of production and secretion of one hormone. It has other cell-
types and of these the alpha cell produces glucagon. Here is one of
the factors which was left out of consideration at the time of the
endocrine balance theory because it was unknown at that point. We
have the adrenal cortex, the pituitary, the adrenal medulla, the
thyroid as the diabetogenic factors, and at that point, glucagon was
only a name given by Murlin to a hyperglycemic factor discovered in
the 1920's (66). After 1948-50, glucagon began to appear as a
possible diabetogenic factor.

The Other Pancreatic Hormone, Glucagon

The current awareness of glucagon endows the phrase "pancreatic
etiology" of diabetes with a meaning different from the old. The
old phrase simply meant "insulin deficiency" which could only be
proven in the juveniles. The new concept may mean that even though
the insulin level is normal, the presence of an abnormal amount of
glucagon and the interplay on the liver of those two factors may produce a diabetic glucose tolerance.

It has been assumed that the pancreatectomized animal has neither insulin nor glucagon, although the gastro-intestinal tract is
intact and there could be either alpha cells or beta cells or both
scattered along the lining of the gastro-intestinal tract. An alloxanized animal does not have insulin if it is severely alloxanized,
but has abnormally high levels of glucagon. If that is so, then the
alloxanized animal ought to show a much different diabetic state from
the standpoint of sugar excretion, ketosis, etc., than the depancreatized animal which lacks glucagon completely or partially. But
perhaps there is no way of obtaining a <u>deglucagonized</u> animal.

There seems to be a group of immunologically related intestinal
peptides forming the glucagon family. Some of these are not active

biologically, i.e., they are not glycogenolytic. However, it would
seem that a peptide indistinguishable from "pancreatic" glucagon is
secreted by intestinal cells. Thus this glucagon is present in the
depancreatized animal. The whole problem of glucagon secretion and
regulation is at present under intensive study (28).

May I conclude by giving you my prejudices. At present, and
for the foreseeable future, the diagnosis of diabetes in many is
based upon finding "inappropriate hyperglycemia", a phrase first
used by Albert Renold. There seems to be no compelling reason as
to why all patients with this finding should be etiologically uniform. The largest group is that of the non-ketotic, reasonably mild,
obese diabetics. Do these individuals simply have a mild version of
the insulin-lack, ketotic diabetes? I do not see why one is compelled
to assume this view exclusively. I suspect that the diabetes of the
obese could be segregated from other forms of diabetes. Etiologically
this may consist of rather normal secretory behavior of the endocrine
organs, but abnormalities in the peripheral tissues. As yet we do
not understand very much about insulin resistance. There may even
be factors in the pancreas, in addition to glucagon and insulin,
which make for resistance to insulin. With respect to other forms
of diabetes, we have some indirect evidence that there is a disturbance of beta cell function in many, or in a large percentage of diabetics. The evidence is less clear, but accumulating, that there is
some change in alpha cell function in diabetics.

That is the dilemma we face at present.

Chapter II – THE NATURE OF DIABETES

DR. UNGER: I think part of the dilemma that we face may be factitious and a nomenclatural dilemma resulting from inadequate definition of the term "diabetes". This has been argued for decades. Probably within this room we would not all agree on what is "diabetes". If, for example, one defines diabetes mellitus as a disease associated with an increased morbidity and mortality attributable to the specific vascular lesions, one identifies a population entirely different from a group of mildly hyperglycemic elderly persons who live to be 80 or more. We should consider how to subclassify the hyperglycemic states. This, I think is what Dr. Levine was really suggesting at the end of his discussion.

DR. LEVINE: You do not solve an issue by changing the name. In other words, I do not care whether we all agree to call them hyperglycemias, which happens to be simply a chemical fact, or we call all the non-transient hyperglycemias "diabetes". That does not really matter. The dilemma is still present: in some of them you think you know the etiology, and in others you do not have as much proof for the etiology.

DR. UNGER: Well, I think we must recognize all of the clinically visible manifestations of disease, and if we do it becomes difficult to equate a 35 year old blind diabetic with an 80 year old man without any abnormality other than the blood sugar disturbance. To consider such dissimilar patients as suffering from the same disease on the basis of a single laboratory test simply does not make sense to me.

DR. LEVINE: But why should I be compelled to reserve the word "diabetes" for those that have blood vessel diseases and die younger?

DR. UNGER: You should not be compelled to do so, but if on arbitrary _a priori_ grounds you decide that there is a single etiology for diseases that may be quite different but have as a common manifestation "hyperglycemia", then I think you have difficulty in trying to solve etiologic questions when you have not really proven that you are studying a single entity.

DR. WOLF: Don't you think, Roger, that it is dangerous to give categorical significance, for example, to mild or severe tuberculosis?

DR. UNGER: I don't mean to suggest that quantitative differences such as mildness and severity should be the basis of differentiation of etiology. I am referring to qualitative differences. Patients with microangiopathy form a relatively homogenous group

which one can study. On the other hand, the people with hyperglycemia who had absolutely no evidence of microangiopathy and
whose life-span is a little bit greater than normal could, I think,
conveniently be grouped in a separate category, particularly since
we know that with advancing age, insulin responsiveness to glucose
decreases. To consider this as "senile hyperglycemia" is not unreasonable in people who are 80 and have an "abnormal glucose tolerance test", which only means that their tolerance is less than
that of the average younger population. I believe that in studying
the etiology of diabetes, one must attempt to have clinically uniform groups, rather than to take everyone with hyperglycemia. The
same logic should be applied to studies of hypertension or any other
disease.

DR. WILLIAMS: Diabetes is a syndrome with the main components
consisting of (a) biochemical changes, especially with regard to
carbohydrate, lipid, protein and nucleotide metabolism; (b) micro-
scopic and macroscopic alterations in various organs of the body,
consisting especially of a characteristic microangiopathy, precocious atherosclerosis and pancreatic islet disorder; (c) deficient insulin action; (d) increased glucagon action; and (e) clinical manifestations due chiefly to altered hydration and osmolality,
microangiopathies and atherosclerosis. There are tremendous differences among diabetic patients with respect to the extent of development of these various disorders and the time of their manifestations. Often, some of the above mentioned abnormalities are manifested relatively much more than others. Indeed, this is true even
when the indications are strong that a genetic disorder is the
basis for the disease.

Much attention has been directed to the pancreatic islets as
a common cause of diabetes. Among the
many reasons for this are that diabetic
The Cells of the   patients have: (a) abnormalities in the
Pancreatic Islets   structure of their islets, demonstrable
at autopsy, (b) deficient insulin levels in their plasma and pancreas, and deficient insulin action, and (c) hyper-normal levels of
glucagon, under certain conditions. Also, many aspects of diabetes
can be readily produced by removal or destruction of the islets,
especially the beta cells.

Gepts (47,83) found histological changes in the islets that
were distinctly different in the following three categories of diabetic patients: (a) "acute juvenile diabetics" — patients with
pronounced clinical manifestations of diabetes that appeared within a few weeks or months before death; (b) patients with "chronic
juvenile diabetes" — these subjects were known to have had diabetes
for several years; and (c) "elderly diabetics" — ones with a course
of adult-onset diabetes. Of the "acute juvenile diabetics" 68% had
insulitis, consisting of both peri- and intra-insular inflammatory

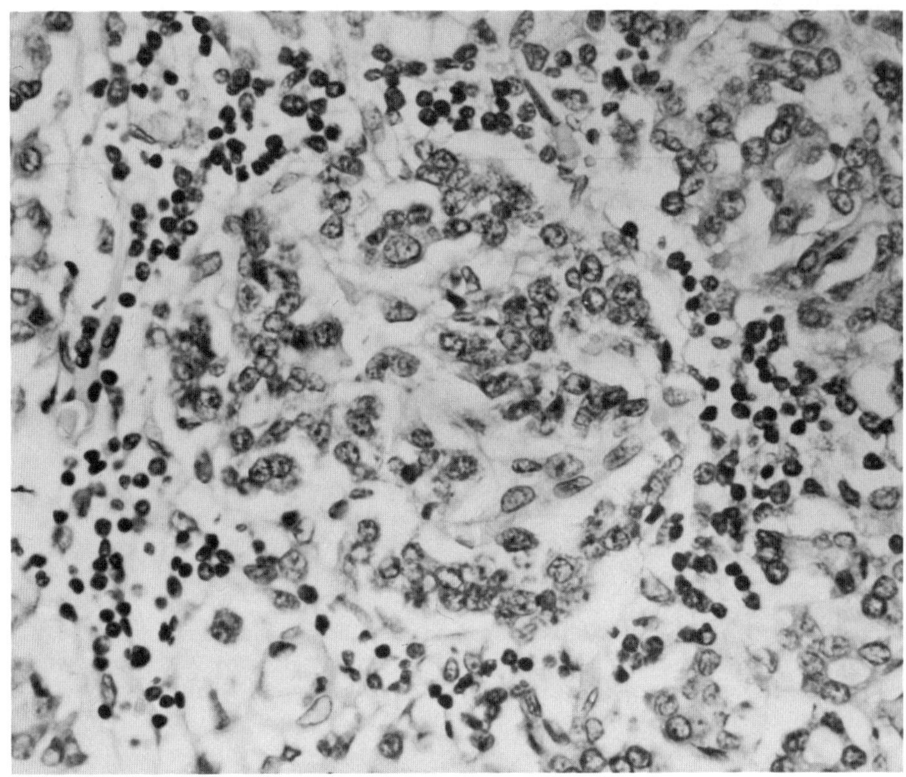

FIG. I. Insulitis showing especially peri-insular
infiltration with lymphocytes. (Section from pancreas
of a girl, age 17, who died from severe ketoacidosis
five days after diagnosis of diabetes and initiation
of insulin treatment. Symptoms appeared four weeks
before death; family history of diabetes.)

infiltrates (Fig. I). Insulitis was not found in "chronic juvenile
diabetes" nor in "elderly diabetics". The type of inflammation with
insulitis was somewhat similar to that produced in animals by the
administration of large amounts of anti-insulin serum, and like that
found in rabbits made diabetic by immunizations with beef insulin.

In "acute juvenile diabetes" there was only about 10% of the
normal number of beta cells. These remaining cells, however, had
manifestations of marked secretory hyperactivity. Many of them
showed nuclear abnormalities. To what extent the hyperplasia of
beta cells was due to compensatory reaction from a deficiency in
insulin produced by the small number of residual cells, and to what
extent it was due to a betacytotrophic effect over a long period is
not known. It is assumed that acute beta cell decompensation was

augmented in a number of instances by episodes of increased body
growth, pregnancy, severe infection, and other stressful effects.
Soon after the acute onset of the clinical manifestations, the
beta cells seemed to decrease progressively, leaving essentially
only alpha cells, a marked decrease in the total size of the islets,
and an accumulation of fibrous tissue. Gepts considered the qualitative lesions, with the exception of those of insulitis, as being
secondary to metabolic disorders in diabetes, and without etiologic
significance.

In the group with "chronic juvenile diabetes" the beta cells
were essentially absent, and the islets consisted chiefly of small
atrophic cells and a significant amount of fibrosis. There was a
decrease in the total number of islets and in the total weight of
the pancreas. In the "elderly diabetics" there was much less
decrease in the quantity of insular tissue; about 50% of the normal number of beta cells was present. Since over 80% of the pancreas can be removed without diabetes, the fact that the number of
beta cells had been reduced 50% should not account for the diabetes,
if they were functioning normally. In this group there was no
insulitis. There was, however, hyalinosis in 41% and fibrosis in
61%. The remaining cells in this elderly group showed relatively
few signs of secretory hyperactivity, despite the numerical deficiency and the associated prolonged hyperglycemia.

Although the studies of Gepts (46,47) are in support of a deficiency in insulin supply once the diabetes is fully manifested,
such observations do not indicate what are the primary changes in
the islets that account for diabetes. Since most instances of
diabetes are presumably on a genetic basis, biochemical alterations
are present before birth. Therefore, it is particularly important
to ascertain the specific nature of the disorder before frank failure
of beta cell activity develops. However, there is remarkable scar-
city of information in this sphere. Scully (122) described a boy,
aged 13, who at the time did not have evidence of diabetes although
he was the son of diabetic parents, but his islets showed considerable hyperplasia. Evans (35) reported a patient who died at the
age of 22 of renal failure. He had been diagnosed as having diabetes
at the age of 9, and sometimes had required as much as 60 units of
insulin daily for control. Autopsy showed increased size of islets
and number of beta cells. Indeed it was estimated that the islets
occupied 10% of the total pancreas (normally they occupy about 2.5%).
A number of important questions arise with respect to the reports
of Scully and Evans. Since Scully's patient can presumably be designated as a prediabetic, it is important to know whether hyperplasia is typical in this stage of development of diabetes. If so,
why does hyperplasia occur? Are there one or more factors that are
stimulating the beta cells to produce insulin excessively? Or does
there tend to be a decrease in net insulin action, with resulting

stimulation of increased beta cell activity? Particularly with
regard to Evans' case the question arises, as he mentioned, as to
whether there was dyshormonogenesis. Or could there be plenty of
insulin but a deficiency in its net activity, with resulting stimulation of the beta cells for increased action? Is there a subnormal
amount of contact inhibition with regard to beta cell growth? Is
there an excess of mesenchymal factor, or of various hormones that
stimulate beta cell proliferation and increased activity?

Since very few observations of the islets have been made in
the prediabetic state, we do not know what are the true changes
during this interval. Assuming that hyperplasia of beta cells is
a characteristic picture, it is especially pertinent to determine
what leads to the marked decrease in the number of beta cells and
to their decreased action. It has long been surmised that constant
marked stimulation of beta cells for several weeks may cause their
exhaustion and degenerative changes. Such has occurred following
the administration of large amounts of sugar to subtotally pancreatectomized animals, or following the administration of large
amounts of growth hormone, or glucocorticoids, or glucagon.

Andersson (4) found that mouse islets cultured in the presence of high glucose concentration (28 mM) showed increased glucose oxidation, but a lower insulin release than islets cultured
at a physiological level (6.7 mM). The high glucose level increased
the rate of conversion of proinsulin to insulin and increased DNA
synthesis, possibly reflecting increased replication of beta cells.
High glucose concentrations also increased the rate of mitosis.
Increased mitotic rate might shorten the life-span of beta cells
to the extent that there is a decrease eventually in the total number of these cells. Logothetopolous (79) concluded that although
beta cells can replicate and increase the volume of islet tissue,
there seems to be a limit in the number of replications; with increase in the rate of replications a state can eventually be obtained when it is either markedly decreased, or stopped. In rats
it was found that the total volume of islet tissue and number of
beta cells were far greater in rats 100 days of age than in those
5 days of age; they were even greater at 480 days. However, the
number of alpha cells increased at a far less rate than that of beta
cells. Moreover, the alpha cells have a lower mitotic activity.
It has not been established whether neogenesis of beta cells from
progenitor stem cells occurs in postnatal life.

DR. SPRITZ: I would like to reinforce the idea that individuals
with the same basic genetic defect, a

The Genetic Component   proclivity toward the development of
hyperglycemic disease, may express the

defect in a variety of ways depending on presently undefined factors
concerned with penetrance. The same is true of the hyperlipidemias.

In affected families one individual may turn up with one form and
another with another. In the case of diabetes I don't think you
can safely single out microvascular lesions as the reliable genetic
marker. A similar phenotype does not necessarily assure the same
genotype.

DR. WOLF: Both you and Roger have made the point that there
are individuals with diabetes who do not have microvascular lesions.
Can we put a timetable on that?

DR. KNOWLES: Many patients are followed with diabetes for
years, even from childhood, without ever developing manifest microvascular disease. On the other hand our methods of diagnosing angiopathy are crude. Our methods of measuring insulin as far as the
dynamics of the 24-hour output are also crude. We have very poor
data on total production rates and secretion rates of insulin in
man, so there may be early chemical defects in insulin production
that we cannot pick up.

DR. SPRITZ: Dr. Knowles has implied that these diabetic
patients represent the same group because they have so little vascular disease. I think it is just as tenable to say that when the
same underlying defect expresses itself in mild form whatever the
basic problem may be, then that is what you see. However, that
doesn't really mean that that's a single pathogenically determined
group by any means.

DR. UNGER: Absolutely. I didn't really mean to make a prior
judgment on that issue. I merely want to advocate that the composition of groups assembled for the purpose of studying etiology
should be a homogeneous one and not a diversified group having in
common only hyperglycemia. That assumes, a priori, that all hyperglycemias are identical and that we will find a single etiology.
I think we have to keep an open mind and study like groups.

DR. SPRITZ: I would argue that we do not know what like groups
are. That like groups in a certain sense may look very different.
All may turn out to have the same underlying defect, but the available evidence does not allow us to say that our present methods of
classification are going to represent homogeneity when we understand
the disease better.

DR. WILLIAMS: I wish to support Dr. Spritz's position with an
example of a diabetic family. FRM, despite frequent examinations
throughout life, was not discovered to have diabetes until the age
of 60. Now at the age of 68, with dietary measures and exercise as
the main therapies, he has relatively little elevation of his plasma
glucose, no clinical indications of microangiopathies, and only a
few of atherosclerosis. However, his son was found to have many

pronounced manifestations of the diabetic process at the age of 5, and died at the age of 31 of diabetic glomerulosclerosis, despite very careful use of diet and insulin. A grandson was found to have diabetes at the age of 5, and is following a course similar to the son. Both the son and the grandson manifested marked deficiency in endogenous insulin action. Since a genetic abnormality was most certainly the cause of diabetes in each of these three people, it is important to consider why the manifestations were so much more marked in the son and grandson. It seems feasible to regard the intensity of the genetic disorder as much more marked in the son and grandson, and consequently that it caused major changes in body physiology much earlier in life. Since it is known that the intensity to which the body reacts to certain abnormalities is far greater in young subjects than in old ones, major differences in clinical manifestations are expected. One of many considerations along this line is the fact that glucagon (increased in diabetes) has far greater lipolytic effect in fat cells of young rats than in older ones (83). Such considerations might account, to some extent, for the differences we see between juvenile-onset diabetes and adult-onset diabetes.

I would like to ask Rachmiel, what are the minimal requirements for designating diabetes? This is something that Dan Portnoy and I had discussions about and he was inclined to say with regard to some of these patients, "Well, tell them that they have hyperglycemia, but don't tell them that they have diabetes." Of course, the next question is, "Well, Doctor, do I or do I not have diabetes?" So I would be interested in hearing what Rachmiel has to say about this.

Prediabetes, chemical diabetes, and diabetes mellitus

DR. LEVINE: I have no answer because there are no independent criteria. But I do think that what we are calling chemical diabetes has to be proven by a normal fasting blood sugar with a small deviation in glucose tolerance. And I must ask if that really belongs in the same category as an individual with a high fasting blood sugar and an abnormal glucose tolerance? It seems to me that we ought to at least separate those two groups.

DR. WILLIAMS: Then it's just a matter of degree, is it not?

DR. LEVINE: Is it just a matter of degree? That is my question. My question is how many individuals — the so-called prediabetic, the potential diabetic, the chemical diabetic — how many of these go on to high fasting glucose levels and symptomatic diabetes?

DR. CAHILL: I think that is a crucial question because, in looking over the clinician's shoulder, I am struck by how many of the patients stay for the rest of their lives at the same level, despite the fact that the diagnosis was made. In other words, a stationary disorder rather than a progressive one.

DR. LEVINE: Right, right.

DR. CAHILL: It is an anomaly, this metabolic disease!

DR. LEVINE: Right, right. And you know, when we heard the Fajans-Conn data (36) we found to our horror that we were not getting the progression we expected. So the question is, are these different disorders?

DR. WOLF: Arthur Mirsky called attention to a paper by O'Sullivan that stated: "48% of those designated as having "chemical diabetes" by the most stringent criteria, and 79% of those diagnosed by more commonly employed but less stringent criteria, show no progression to further carbohydrate decompensation over a period of 10 years. Furthermore, an earlier study revealed that 54% of a group of young nonpregnant women with "chemical diabetes" exhibited normal tolerance curves within two years thereafter." (104,105)

DR. WILLIAMS: I would like to hear Dr. Levine's views on the other facets of the syndrome.

DR. WOLF: You mean the microvascular lesions?

DR. LEVINE: You mean at some time one can have advanced microvascular disease with normal glucose curves at least for a period of time?

DR. WILLIAMS: Yes.

DR. LEVINE: Yes. Some years ago I had a patient, a 42-year old single woman, whose physician referred her to me because he saw retinopathy and she complained of spots in front of her eyes. Her blood sugar was normal. Her glucose tolerance was normal too. It was at that point that he called me and I took her into our Metabolic Unit in Chicago and we did nine glucose tolerance tests in as many weeks. Eight of these tests were normal and the ninth slightly abnormal; a chemical diabetes. She had bilateral, diffuse retinopathy, a heavy albuminuria and she showed the Kimmelstiel-Wilson lesion by renal biopsy, the typical nodular Kimmelstiel-Wilson picture, retention of BUN, etc. She then went to the Mayo Clinic, where she was seen in the Opthalmology Department, who told her she had not taken care of her diabetes. She was sent to the Diabetes group who could not make a decision of diabetes. But, and I emphasize this, her mother died in diabetic coma; one sister had an amputation and was a known diabetic. She herself weighed 200 pounds when she was 20 years old. So she was scared of the whole situation and reduced her weight to around 109 pounds for the rest of the time and did not manifest any overt disturbances on the metabolic side but only showed this disturbance in the eyes and kidneys.

I don't know what this teaches us; perhaps that by dint of severe metabolic deprivation one can reduce the glucose aspects of the disorder down to a minimum without abolishing the capillary disorder. It may simply mean that if for twenty years you treat someone in order to reduce the blood sugar down to normal, you cannot expect that you will stop or abolish the capillary syndrome. On the other hand, I don't know that if she had allowed herself an increased food intake and greater weight at age 20, whether she would not have been dead from renal insufficiency in 2 to 4 years, rather than 20 to 25 years. We simply do not know.

DR. WOLF: One of our guest medical students, Charles Rost, raised the question, "What can be said about heredity in diabetes? Is the implication a single gene or a multiple allele?"

The pattern of
Inheritance

DR. SPRITZ: I think you can make the one negative statement: In the families that were studied none of the standard Mendelian transmission criteria are well supported.

DR. LEVINE: But I must hasten to add that Albert Renold might say there are genetic forms of hyperglycemia in rodents, some of which are well known genetically, and others not so well. The ob-ob animal has a single recessive gene characterized by a mild non-ketotic diabetes, hyperglycemia with obesity and tremendous amounts of insulin cruising around in the blood and yet, has insulin resistance. There is another variant called DB-DB, which is also a single gene recessive character but on another chromosome. These animals start out looking remarkably like the ob-ob but then the symptoms get worse, the animals become ketotic and develop insulin-requiring diabetes. There are other forms of genetically segregated rodents that have diabetes in various forms; some have hyperinsulin-ism and others do not. These are rodents (gerbils, spiny mice, etc.) of one kind or another. Also, there are diabetic primates (baboons, etc.). So there is no doubt that in nature there are some single gene defects and multi-genic types of non-transient hyperglycemia with or without obesity, with or without ketosis. On the basis of these findings, at least it is not too uncomfortable to suppose that if one accepts the whole gamut of hyperglycemia as a syndrome that one could have multiple etiologies in multiple types of inheritance. Steinberg used to call diabetes a disease with variable recessive penetrance (133). Now we have given up calling it anything. There is one Rumanian worker who, on the basis of his large series of cases, says diabetes is a Mendelian dominant (106).

DR. SPRITZ: I agree that in human diabetes there appears to
be an important genetic component. If that is true, we would like
to understand exactly what is transmitted genetically. The rest of
the picture represents non-genetic modifications or external modifications related to when the disease expresses itself, whether or
not certain aspects, such as microvascular lesions, appear. It is
even possible that auxiliary genes besides the ones we are talking
about, may precipitate the clinical onset of the disease and the
manner in which it is expressed. The best genetic information we
have suggests that the clinical manifestations of a disease can
vary in different people and still have the same genetic basis.

DR. WOLF: Familial aggregation is a safer term.

DR. LEVINE: In a diabetic family such as Dr. Williams described earlier, you could also have an 80 year old with a small
disturbance in glucose tolerance who is picked up because of a one
plus glycosuria at one time. You tend to say these people are all
the same. They may not be. Even if they have a gene called diabetes
the 80 year old one may not have any genetic tendency at all. He
may simply be peculiar in pancreatic function, like all of us will
be at one time.

We know that in some people we will not diagnose diabetes until
they are 60, even though we visualize that the disorder is on the
basis of a genetic disturbance. If it is genetic, they are born
with a biochemical disorder. They cannot have such a high incidence
of the microvascular disease without having a biochemical disturbance for many years.

EDITORIAL NOTE

Since the Colloquium a paper by Tattersall (135) and one by
Tattersall and Fajans (136) reported studies of the pattern of inheritance of mild maturity onset type diabetes occurring in young
people as contrasted with that observed in the classical juvenile
onset diabetes mellitus. The evidence indicated an autosomal dominant pattern for the mild maturity-onset type. The number of affected
offspring was considerably fewer in the juvenile onset type suggesting genetic heterogeneity or a less significant genetic role. In
this connection it is interesting that Huff and associates have
reported a cluster of cases of juvenile onset diabetes following
closely on a community-wide outbreak of influenza (60). They
reviewed other published evidence of a possible viral etiology but
were unable to inculpate any particular virus in their own cases.
Other studies going back more than 100 years have suggested a link
between diabetes and mumps. Coxsackie virus infections have also

been correlated with the onset of juvenile diabetes. Perhaps a
genetic predilection may be triggered by viral damage to the pancreas or to the mechanisms that regulate pancreatic endocrine function.

DR. WILLIAMS: We do know that the diabetic picture is produced by various types of viruses such
Precipitating   as the Coxsackie virus, mumps and there
Factors   are others. I might mention, parenthe-
tically, that one student who was work-
ing with me who had no history or evidence of diabetes in his parents
or anyone in his family, developed a very acute onset of diabetes
about a week or ten days after a bout of the flu. He had an elevated Coxsackie virus level. Reports are appearing with increased
frequency suggesting that diabetes in some patients may result from
a viral infection. The Coxsackie virus and mumps virus are etiologic agents. After injecting encephalomyocarditis virus into mice,
Wellman et al. (144) demonstrated it in pancreas, and that there
resulted disruption of islet cell architecture, beta cell necrosis,
beta cell degranulation and mononuclear cell infiltration. Then
there was a deficiency in pancreatic insulin and an increase in
blood glucose. Although it is clearly conceivable that diabetes
can be produced in an individual instance from a viral infection,
there are two questions in particular that loom strongly, namely
(a) could such lead to genetic alterations with appearance of diabetes in succeeding generations, and (b) could it also lead to the
characteristic microangiopathy in succeeding generations of patients
with diabetes? The answer to both of these questions must include
an affirmative possibility. For such, however, it is necessary to
have genetic alterations in the germ plasm.

I have some information that is worthy of at least consideration along this line. It is not work
Experimental Diabetes –   with viruses, but rather with alloxan.
Chemical influences on   These are studies in rabbits, guinea
Genetic equipment   pigs and in rats where one produced
alloxan diabetes, and in some instances
this was done in the females and in some others it was in the males,
then they bred these animals in a great variety of ways. Alloxan
was also given to succeeding generations. It was found that after
about five generations, a fair number of animals developed spontaneous diabetes although those animals never received alloxan. The
incidence of diabetes was just as high when the paternal diabetics
were bred with a non-diabetic mother as it was when both parents
were diabetic. The incidence of diabetes in succeeding generations
was not as high if those animals were treated for four weeks or
more before the breeding. We should ask in this connection whether
or not the alloxan not only damaged the beta cell of the animal to
which it was administered, but also its germ cell, because we know

that alloxan can damage the lung and many other tissues. The mere
having of diabetes in the mother may bring about certain biochemical changes in the germ plasm which will lead to a permanent genetic disorder.

Spergel et al. (128) used subdiabetogenic doses of alloxan
and only gave the compound to the original parents. Glucose tolerance tests showed deterioration with successive breeding of rats.
In both studies the need for a diabetic environment was eliminated
by the fact that the descendents of diabetic fathers acquired diabetes as frequently as the descendents of the two diabetic parents.
Chromosomal descriptions were not reported, but it is possible that
there were transmissable changes in regulator genes concerned with
glucose metabolism. Alterations in this metabolism might also arise
through several mechanisms, including the possible alterations that
led to the development of autoimmune disease in each of the succeeding generations. Incidentally we know that sand rats, in their
natural environment, do not have diabetes but when brought in the
laboratory and given a usual diet, diabetes occurs in some.

DR. CAHILL: Just to summarize, I think there is more and
more evidence to support the idea that there is a genetic instabil-
ity in the tissues in the diabetic kindred and on top of that is
added something else. I think that Marvin Siperstein is right,
that there is probably some primary basic abnormality. I think
that Vracko is right. Because I think there is some diffuse cellular process, but at least in the kidney this is markedly accelerated
by the diabetes itself. That is why the Danes (Hansen, for example)
showed that you cannot really detect any severe abnormality in the
kidney early in the juvenile diabetic, but two or three years later
you begin to see it (Work in progress).

Now comes the question, does the glucose molecule have anything to do with the abnormal glyco-
protein accumulation in diabetes? Cer-
Glucose as an   tainly this is one of the reasons we
Etiologic agent   are here today. We are here to find
out how much is inherent (how much is genetic) and how much is
added on by the biochemical abnormalities that take place in the
diabetic. If you want to know my answer ... it is both! Can
glucose itself, when present in high concentration, initiate any
kind of metabolic alteration? Here is another piece of obscurity
which was really discovered in the mid-1960s when a group of hema-
tologists working on hemoglobinopathies, doing electrophoresis,
came across a couple of diabetics. To their surprise, they found
there was a fast-moving component that certain diabetics had in
the hemoglobin. Fig. II illustrates the work of Trivelli and
Ranney (137). About one-quarter of juvenile diabetics will have
a significant increase in a component called the A-1-C component.

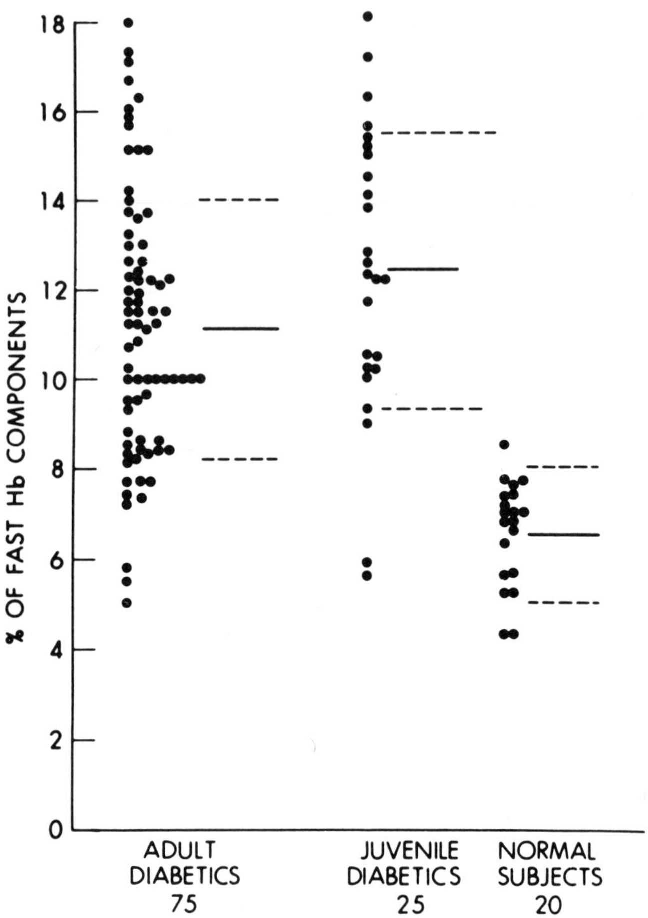

FIG. II. (After Trivelli, Ranney, Lai).

This hemoglobin moves abnormally rapidly, electrophoretically. One
cannot diagnose diabetes electrophoretically by doing an electrophoresis of hemoglobin since there is a lot of overlap between
fractions. Originally it was thought that this might be an independent expression of the gene, but when looked at in mild diabetics,
there is even more overlap. The correlation with glucose is poor
but if you realize that the red cells have been around for a month
or two and were synthesized at a slow and variable rate, to corre-
late the degree of carbohydrate abnormality on day X at the same
time that the blood was drawn, is meaningless since the red cell
was made days to weeks previously. It is an interesting observation but it is a benign process because it apparently does nothing

to 2-3 diphosphoglycerate or to the Bohr effect. Like many of the
inherited hemoglobinopathies it is a benign alteration. The real
question is why is it a fast moving hemoglobin? It is fast moving
because, to the surprise of the hematologist, hemoglobin is a
glycoprotein and it has a small per cent of carbohydrate stuck on
to it, very similar to one of the carbohydrate structures on basement membrane. So, here you have the bone marrow in a given individual which synthesizes an excess of an abnormal glycoprotein in
the presence of diabetes.

DR. SPRITZ: What lends the mobility to it?

DR. CAHILL: I believe it is because of a sialic acid on the
terminal end which adds a negative charge to the molecule.

DR. WOLF: And you say that the identical twin of the diabetic would be in the normal range?

DR. CAHILL: Yes, that is what all the evidence suggests.
Actually I do not know about the identical twin, but the prediabetic
and the mild diabetic without hyperglycemia for a long period of
time, when tested, do not have this alteration. In other words,
one has to have a degree of hyperglycemia and obviously one has to
have prolonged uncontrolled diabetes.

DR. LEVINE: 85% of the hemoglobin in the diabetic does not
have this extra molecule.

DR. CAHILL: Yes, you are correct. Also this component is
present in the normal up to about 6%. It is just increased in the
diabetic.

DR. LEVINE: I am skeptical because many workers have been
unable to identify the molecular abnormality as characteristic of
diabetes.

DR. CAHILL: That is most important, if that is true.

DR. LEVINE: Someone has to do a big study before it can be
accepted. Dr. Ranney is now at San Diego and has been talking with
our group about doing this.

DR. KNOWLES: Does this thing increase with age?

DR. CAHILL: I do not know. At this point I have not seen any
age correlations.

DR. WILLIAMS: Do you know of data on any pre-diabetics with
respect to their glucagon secretion?

DR. UNGER: We studied a group in cooperation with Stuart
Soeldner in which the Boston pre-diabetics were compared to the
group of Dallas controls. These were individuals who were recruited
through the newspapers without any known family history of diabetes,
but had at least six immediate relatives, such as brothers, sisters,
uncles and aunts. We tried to match them demographically and socio-
economically. The data obtained are very hard to interpret. The
only differences that we found were with regard to their response to
arginine. In the control group there was an age-related increase in
the glucagon response to arginine, whereas in the diabetic group
there was no such correlation with age. Right now we are in the process of doing a study in the Pima Indian Group with Drs. Bennett and
Aronoff in Arizona, in the hope that better matching of controls
will permit an evaluation.

DR. CAHILL: Soeldner collected a dozen or so identical twins,
ranging in age from 10 to 25 or 30 (in preparation). In those individuals we could demonstrate absolutely no abnormality of insulin
release or glucagon, and if present, the abnormality occurred in a
very small number. They were identical twins of a known juvenile
diabetic. In one case of triplets, two were normal and one was a
juvenile diabetic. The two normals had no insulin delay. Subsequently, the second of the two siblings of the triplets ultimately
developed juvenile diabetes (21).

DR. WOLF: You mean that someone you had studied previously
and in whom no abnormality was found, subsequently developed the
juvenile diabetes.

DR. BERLE: In how many years?

DR. CAHILL: Yes. We studied these triplets at frequent inter-
vals. After perfectly normal carbohydrate and insulin and glucagon
kinetics, the second triplet went on to develop juvenile-type diabetes.

DR. WOLF: I would like to ask Dr. Levine to expand on the concept of depletion or wearing out of beta
Depletion of   cells which has been very prominent in
Secretory Cells   postgraduate courses and in literature
reviews. Is there any evidence in the
pancreas, or indeed in any other tissue, that excessive stimulation
may result in depletion?

DR. LEVINE: I would say that there is little convincing evidence for overstimulation of the pancreas by glucose or otherwise,
leading to an exhaustion of the pancreas. On the other hand back
in the 30's Lukens and Long produced hemorrhagic damage in the pancreas in cats by administration of large amounts of glucose but

there was never a clear production of permanent diabetes (80).
In some animals diabetes can be produced by prolonged administration
of tremendous amounts of growth hormone. Adult dogs but not pups,
cats or pregnant dogs are susceptible to this technique. In the
adult rat, growth hormone will not even produce transient diabetes.
However, in humans if you have the spontaneous occurrence of acromegaly, you will get from about 60-70% patients (with acromegaly)
with proliferation of the islets and stimulation for as long as it
goes on without exhaustion; but about 25-30% will become diabetic.
This is a point that Rolf Luft makes: acromegalics who have a
prompt insulin response to glucose will never exhaust; acromegalics
who do exhaust are the ones that have the earmarks of an early diabetes; that is, a non-prompt or delayed response to glucose.

DR. SPRITZ: What about the DB mouse? It goes through a hyperplastic phase histologically, a high insulin phase and then a low
insulin phase, at the time of death.

DR. LEVINE: Yes, but the high insulin phase in DB mice is no
higher than in the ob-ob which does not exhaust. However, there
must be something genetic in that they cannot maintain this high
glucose level without developing diabetes.

DR. UNGER: We are revealing our amazing ignorance about the
human diabetic pancreas because we
Beta cell Histology   really do not know the number of islets,
in Humans   what their replication rate is, what
the death rate of beta cells is, the
number of cells per islet, or whether there are any identifiable
lesions. All we know is based on studies of plasma hormone concentrations.

DR. SPRITZ: We don't really know the role of aging and increased intolerance to glucose and its effect on the beta cell and
the pancreas. Is there a loss of beta cell units with age? Do we
know anything about the morphologic changes in the beta cell associated with increasing glucose intolerance in aging subjects? For
example, has there been a count of beta cells? Do we know whether
a 70 year old has as many beta cells as a person had before? Has
anybody done that work?

DR. ORCI: Up to the present there has been no morphological
analysis of the number of beta cells in the human. Only now are
these studies being undertaken because the technique of morphological study is very discouraging but it is being undertaken now. It
has not been very satisfactory.

DR. LEVINE: How do you get the samples in the human?

DR. ORCI: Oh, not in the human! However, we can do these things at autopsy.

DR. LEVINE: Yes, but that is after years and years of diabetes. What we want to know is what is the picture regarding the beta cell when the glucose tolerance deviates and becomes abnormal.

DR. ORCI: Well, some of these autopsies can be done on individuals who died as a result of an accident and in a situation like this we have to effect a compromise.

DR. WILLIAMS: I have never seen any report of studies of beta cells in humans. I don't know how you can satisfactorily get the beta cells out unless you remove the whole pancreas. However, in rats it has been reported that the number of islets and the number of beta cells increases with age. After five days, 100 days and 480 days there was a distinct increase in both the number of islets and the number of beta cells. The slope in the rise of the beta cells was far greater than the rise in the alpha cells, although they increased too. In regard to man, Sulzer showed that aged people given a high intake of food for at least one week displayed a glucose tolerance test typical of people at age 50. Some would infer that high caloric intake yields a more sensitive "set" in the islets so that they respond more briskly with insulin production to the increased glucose intake. Normally the number of insulin receptors appears to decrease with age, but maintaining a limited food intake may restore insulin receptor activity to normal.

DR. CAHILL: As Dr. Williams indicated, it is pretty clear that insulin, and in fact all peptide hormones, work by their capacity to bind to receptors that are on a cell membrane. These set up some secondary process inside the cell as well as alterations in membrane. As far as insulin is concerned, every cell that has been tested in the body has insulin receptors. In fact, recently Victor Conard of Brussels, has shown that if one takes the marine plant, acetabularia, chemically speaking one can define insulin receptors on its membrane (24). So it appears that all living tissues including brain cells (which have not been examined for this as far as I know) have insulin receptors. Perhaps even oak trees have some insulin receptors on their cell membrane! The specificity as to what this means can be questioned. It is interesting that lymphocytes according to Jesse Roth and others (119), have insulin receptors, but it is almost impossible to demonstrate an insulin effect either in terms of glucose uptake, glycogen synthesis, CO_2 formation or fatty acid synthesis in the lymphocyte (18).

The Actions of Insulin

So the specificity of cells is not a function of their recep-

tors but is rather what happens after the receptor has been acted
upon. Again, just two minutes of history. I was taught in medical
school, and I was just at that flex point before the Huddlestein,
Goldstein, Levine publication came out, that what insulin did was
to alter the phosphorylation capacity inside the cell by way of the
Cori hypothesis; that when one mashed up a muscle and measured its
phosphorylation capacity inside the cell, in the insulin deficient
animal, this was decreased. However, if you gave the animal insulin for a period of time, it was returned back to normal. Then came
the hypothesis of an antidiabetic effect involving the pituitary,
etc., etc., etc. But it is interesting now that the whole cycle
seems to be turned around, because there is no question that muscle
cells in a diabetic animal display phosphorylation capacity. This
is because hexokinase is down and will not go into the isozome form.
So there is no question but that insulin does exert an intracellular
enzyme effect. One can take a whole list of enzymes some 40 or
50 which are demonstrably altered by the presence of insulin. There
are, for example, glucose 6-phosphate dehydrogenase and fatty acid
synthetase, glycogen synthetase, and so on. So insulin has some
second messenger which alters many processes including processes on
the cell membrane as well as many enzymes. One has to remember
that there are certain temporal sequences whereby insulin works.

DR. CAHILL: I want to talk now about the influence of glucose
on the cell membrane. It is interesting
that when I joined the Department of
Glucose as a
Metabolic Regulator
Biochemistry at Harvard about eight
years after the Goldstein-Levine publi-
cations, it was freely extrapolated by most physiologists that all
cells responded to insulin by augmented glucose transport. The
pendulum had swung so far with Dr. Levine's persuasive character
that every cell in the body, except liver cells, was insulin responsive and that what insulin did was to tell all cells to take up
glucose. We now know, or are fairly certain, that this hypothesis
really applies to only two tissues in the body, muscle and fat. If
you look at any other cell in the body you cannot demonstrate a
facilitation of glucose entry by insulin. The brain cell, for
example, has a very highly stereospecific glucose entry system,
recognizing only glucose and a few minor modifications of glucose
such as mannose, galactose, 3-0-methyl glucose, also a few pentoses.
But if you change the sugar around any further the brain cell will
not recognize the substance. But the Ymax is so rapid or so marked
in all cells of the body that essentially, glucose equilibration
between extracellular and intracellular fluids takes place, since
the rate at which glucose can cross the cell membrane far surpasses
the capacity of glucose phosphorylation. This has been shown by
us (although not published), and by others, when tissues such as
the kidney, spleen or skin are analyzed. In fact, every cell in
the body seems to have no problem in letting glucose enter with the

exception of muscle and adipose tissue. This makes sense. Muscle
and adipose cells are the two tissues that have to be signaled after
a large meal to take up and remove the excess glucose which is
coming in.

The endothelial cells always "sees" the ambient concentration
of glucose throughout the body. This is also true for the central
nervous system. So what I am really saying is that all cells in
the body, except for muscle and adipose tissue, "see" the same concentration of glucose as is present in the circulation or a concentration close to it. Therefore, the next question is, whether
or not glucose is bad for the cells if it should get too high.

First we have to examine whether the glucose molecule can
itself do anything other than act as a substrate, say, for certain
enzymes such as sorbitol formation, or phosphorylation by hexokinase
and glucokinase. Gerry Hers has some data on the enzymes involved
in glycogen synthesis and breakdown (27). One or more of these
enzymes are directly affected by the insulin molecule and this is
the first time, to my knowledge, that glucose as a molecule itself
can work as a signal.

DR. LEVINE: Dr. Cahill, does Gerry Hers still maintain that
insulin is not necessary for this allosteric reaction?

DR. CAHILL: Insulin is necessary for another step in the
glycogen synthesis reaction, in other words we have a summation of
glucose and insulin. There is no question that insulin by lowering cyclic AMP, increases the activity of the glycogen synthetase
complex. But what I am saying is that, in addition to that total
activity, there is a greater rate of glycogen-synthesis activity
than one can explain unless one invokes an allosteric activation
of the system by the glucose molecule itself. So Hers feels that
whenever the glucose is elevated inside the liver cell, it augments
incorporation of uridinediphosphoglucose into glycogen. This means
at least that the glucose molecule can have biochemical activity
of its own. I believe emphatically that it is also the glucose
molecule that stimulates insulin release from the beta cell. It
is not a sequela to glucose metabolism. In other words, I am on
the Matschinsky side not on the Randle side, because I believe that
the speed and the extremely high stereospecificity for glucose to
initiate insulin release, as well as the failure of fructose, which
is readily metabolized by the beta cells, to stimulate insulin release. This suggests an allosteric recognition of the glucose
molecule by some receptor proteins. If glucose as a molecule inside
a cell can alter at least one known enzymatic reaction, then it may
be able to alter others. I am throwing this out as a sort of teaser,
more or less. In summary, let us leave this by saying that the
glucose molecule itself, which is equilibrated with blood glucose

concentration in all cells except muscle and adipose tissue, is able to exert probably at least one metabolic effect on the synthesis of a polysaccharide, glycogen, and there may be many more we don't know about.

DR. UNGER: We first became interested in the possibility that the alpha and beta cells and islets of Langerhans function, not as independent neighbors in the sense that some of the cells of the hypophysis function, but rather as a single, coordinated if not coupled functional unit designed to control the flux of key nutrients into and out of cells in accordance with supply and demand. This view was based on the remarkable qualitative relationship observed between the relative concentrations of the two hormones and the known, measured, or suspected need for a particular movement of nutrients. When the need of the organism was for breakdown of macro-molecules so that the important nutrients may be surrendered, the relative concentrations of insulin to glucagon was invariably low. Conversely, when synthesis of macromolecules was appropriate, the relative concentration of insulin to glucagon was always high. More recently there has been additional support for alpha-beta cell coup-ling. Dr. Orci has demonstrated an anatomical basis for inter-cellular communication between alpha and beta cells in the islets of Langerhans in the form of junctional complexes.

Let me first address myself to Dr. Levine's question: "Why is there a need for glucagon? Why won't the changes in the concentra-tion of insulin by itself do everything that is needed? Why do we need a push-pull Sherringtonian system?". I think the answer to those questions is this: This is the only way that one can maintain glucose concentration within the very narrow range that normally prevails in healthy individuals. For example, Fig. III shows that during the infusion of an amino acid such as arginine which stimulates both hormones, glucose turnover changes substantially but glucose concentration stays very constant. Insulin has increased the out-flow of glucose from the extracellular space but glucagon is replac-ing it by raising hepatic glucose production so as to prevent hypo-glycemia from the insulin. Very elegant studies from Toronto by Cherrington and Vranic indicate that under similar circumstances glucose turnover rises up to 70% but glucose concentration stays relatively constant. Insulin changes alone could not achieve this; if insulin should rise without glucagon, glucose would fall. More-over, the metabolic options provided by the bi-hormonal system would be lacking. It is, for example, possible for the liver to produce glucose without at the same time increasing lipolysis, because glu-cagon can increase glucose production without a decline in insulin. Similarly it is possible, thanks to the bi-hormonal arrangement, to produce glucose and at the same time incorporate amino acids into protein. This would not be possible if insulin change were the only regulatory control of these functions. At the opposite extreme is the "endocrine pancreatectomy" produced by somatostatin, a hormone which has been shown by Goodner's group in Seattle and several other

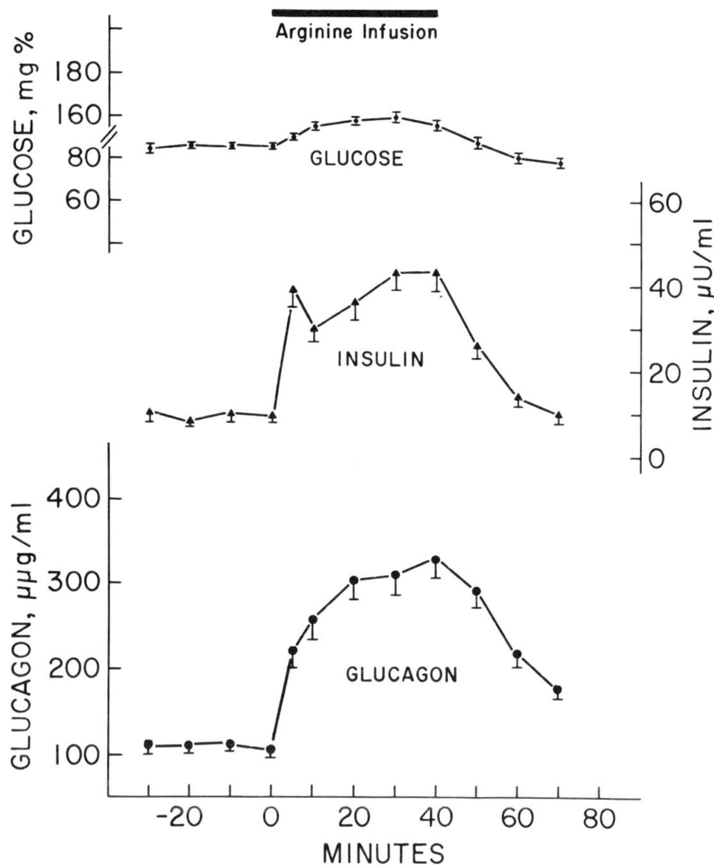

FIG. III. The glucagon and insulin response
to arginine in normal subjects.

groups, to inhibit both insulin and glucagon (52). There is very
little change in glucose concentration when both hormones are de-
pressed and one would predict a fall in glucose turnover with, once
again, very little change in glucose concentration. The tenacity
with which glucose concentration is maintained within the normal
range is, I think relevant to one of our dilemmas in diabetes,
namely, is gluco-regulation very important to health? If the organism is continually in the process of synthesizing macromolecules
or breaking them down - the macromolecules such as glycogen and
triglycerides, being synthesized for the purpose of cell growth
and replication, for the enzymatic machinery, and for energy storage - the insulin-glucagon antagonism may provide a vital regulatory
mechanism (see Table 1). In the case of the liver, for example,

TABLE 1

DEMONSTRATED OPPOSITION ON COMMON
TARGETS: INSULIN VS. GLUCAGON

TARGET	EFFECT	INSULIN	GLUCAGON
Liver	Glycogenesis	↑	↓
	Glycogenolysis	↓	↑
	Gluconeogenesis	↓	↑
	VLDL Secretion	↑	↓
	Lysosome Formation	↓	↑
Fat	Lipolysis	↓	↑

the two hormones balance each other with respect to glycogenesis
and glycogenolysis. A high concentration of insulin relative to
glucagon would promote glycogenesis in excess of glycogenolysis,
would oppose gluconeogenesis and increase the secretion of very
low density lipoproteins (VLDL) by the liver. It would also oppose
hepatic lysosome formation. And I could add that recent data from
Leffert in La Jolla (75) and from Price in New York (111) suggests
that a high concentration of insulin relative to glucagon is essential for DNA synthesis in quiescent liver tissue; if one decreases
the relative concentration of insulin to glucagon, one inhibits the
regeneration of liver in partially hepatectomized animals. So at
every level, wherever they have a common target tissue, the two
hormones appear to counter balance one another.

I mentioned before the anatomical evidence which Dr. Orci had
provided to support the notion that the anatomical proximity bridges
between alpha and beta cells might possibly enter into their coordinated function. In Dr. Orci's presentation, beginning on page 62
he shows that the tight junctions appear to be as anastomosing
ridges, and gap junctions appear as hexagonally arranged particles.
Gap junctions may be the site of electrical coupling between cells,

which would explain coordinated secretory activity of these cells
that are not well explained by external stimulation alone. We
would then choose to view the alpha-beta cell couple as having
such communications and as constituting a bi-hormonal functional
unit capable of directing the key nutrients into macromolecular
synthesis when precursors of such molecules are available in the
form of diet, or when they are not available, or when the need for
fuel increases, appropriate function of this coupled unit promotes
the catabolism of these macromolecules for energy production. And
as we will attempt to show, the primary control mechanism for secretion by these cells are the circulating arterial nutrients themselves.

DR. LEVINE: If you add a set of nutrients as the signals which
stimulate either the alpha or the beta into operation or inhibit
one while stimulating the other, then what is the need for communication between alpha and beta itself? This is in accordance with
your previous description.

DR. UNGER: Well, first of all, there is a remarkable (as we
will see a little bit later) quantitative precision as to what is
released by these structures. Secondly, these cells are not functioning synchronously, yet their net hormonal output is so remarkably titrated that it becomes a little difficult to explain without some sort of coordinated orchestration. It has been shown that
particles, compounds of a molecular weight of less than 500, such
as fluorescein can pass through such cell membranes without enter-
ing the intercellular spaces.

DR. ORCI: If you injected into one cell, fluorescein, which
has a molecular weight of about 500,
The Alpha Beta   you can then follow the trans-location
Cell Couple   of this dye as it passes through an ad-
joining cell, without leakage into the
intercellular spaces. And this happens only where both cells are
coupled by such membrane specialization which is the gap junction.

DR. SPRITZ: This implies that cells adjacent to each other
really "see" what goes on in one another.

DR. UNGER: Once again I would like to stress the flexibility
of the alpha-beta cell couple in normal individuals in relation
to the need and availability of energy yielding fuels (see Fig. IV).
When the fuels are available, it is the function of the normal
alpha-beta cell couple to operate in such a way as to provide enough
insulin relative to glucagon to permit the synthesis of these precursors into the large molecules. On the other hand, when these
fuels are not available, or when the need for fuel increases, it is
the function of the normal alpha-beta cell couple to maintain a

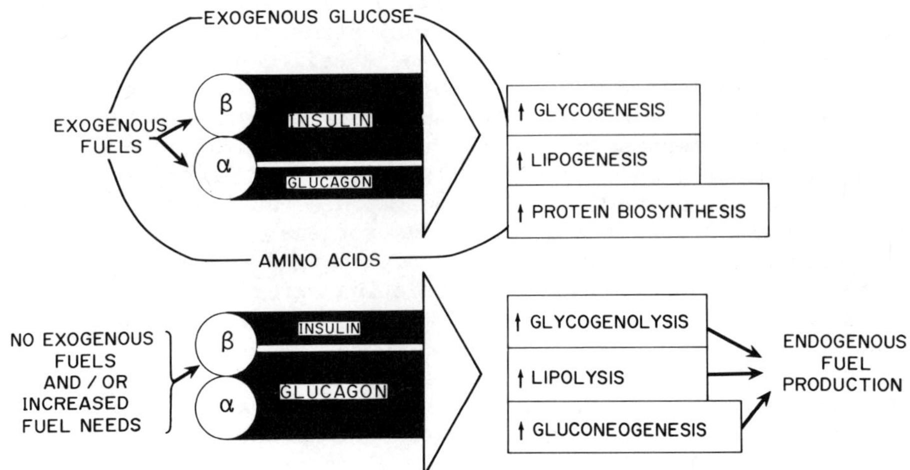

FIG. IV. The comparison of insulin and glucagon secretion and the resulting effect on various metabolic processes during an abundance of exogenous fules and/or increased fuel needs.

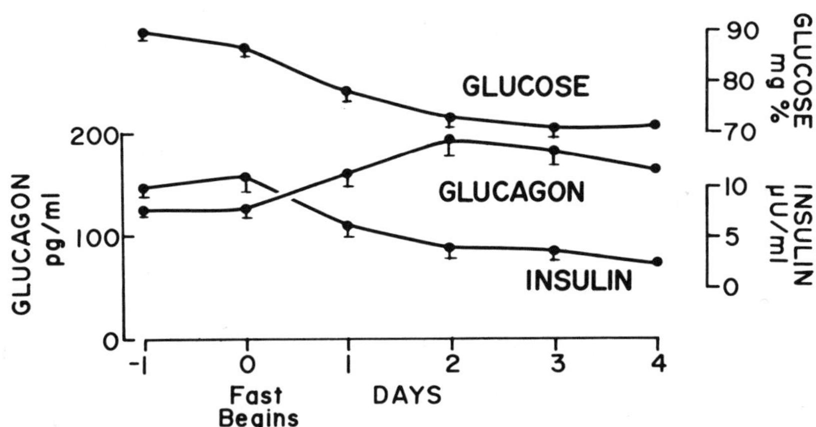

FIG. V. The effect of total starvation upon insulin and glucagon levels in normal volunteers.

concentration of insulin relative to glucagon which will permit
the breakdown of glycogen and fat and when necessary, the very
parsimonious surrendering of amino acids derived from endogenous
protein to permit endogenous glucose production.

As I said before, one of the things that struck us in physiological studies was the fact that the relative concentration of the
two hormones appeared to decline as need for endogenous fuel production rose, as during starvation or severe exercise, for example
(see Fig. V). Under these circumstances insulin-glucagon ratio
was invariably low. During starvation it is low because of a reciprocal fall in insulin and a corresponding rise in glucagon. In
severe exercise, by contrast, the same low ratio is observed but it
was the result, not so much of a fall in insulin, as of a marked
increase in glucagon (see Fig. VI). Similarly, as one increases
the glucose availability, and decreases the need for glucose, one
observes an ever rising concentration of insulin relative to glucagon (see Fig. VII). During violent exercise to the point of
collapse, there is an extremely low insulin-glucagon ratio. The
basal insulin-glucagon ratio is 2 or 3 and at the point of collapse
would fall to 0.2 or 0.3. As a consequence of this, the tremendous
rise in glucagon results in sufficient endogenous glucose production
to meet the increased utilization of glucose and prevent hypoglycemia. This hormonal response appears to be mediated by adrenergic
stimulation. As Dr. Porte has shown, (110) increased adrenergic
activity will reduce insulin, which permits the hyperglucagonemia
to increase glucose production without glucose loss into insulin
dependent tissues.

DR. LEVINE: Roger, how did the original glucagon secretion
rise? In other words, to what stimulus was the alpha cell responding?

DR. UNGER: I suspect epinephrin because you can block it with
adrenergic blocking agents, virtually or completely.

DR. LEVINE: And, therefore, the epinephrin response is not
due to low blood sugar either and, if so, then what is it due to?

DR. UNGER: This must be centrally controlled. I do not know
the mechanism. But the glucagon response to exercise closely re-
sembles the response to stress in hypovolemic shock, whether due to
infection or trauma — this is what you see. Thus, insulin is fixed
irrespective of glucose concentration and glucagon is high irrespective of glucose concentration.

DR. SPRITZ: To achieve a greater increase in production of
glucose by the liver and utilization by muscle, in the presence
of a low level of insulin, would you not have to supply something

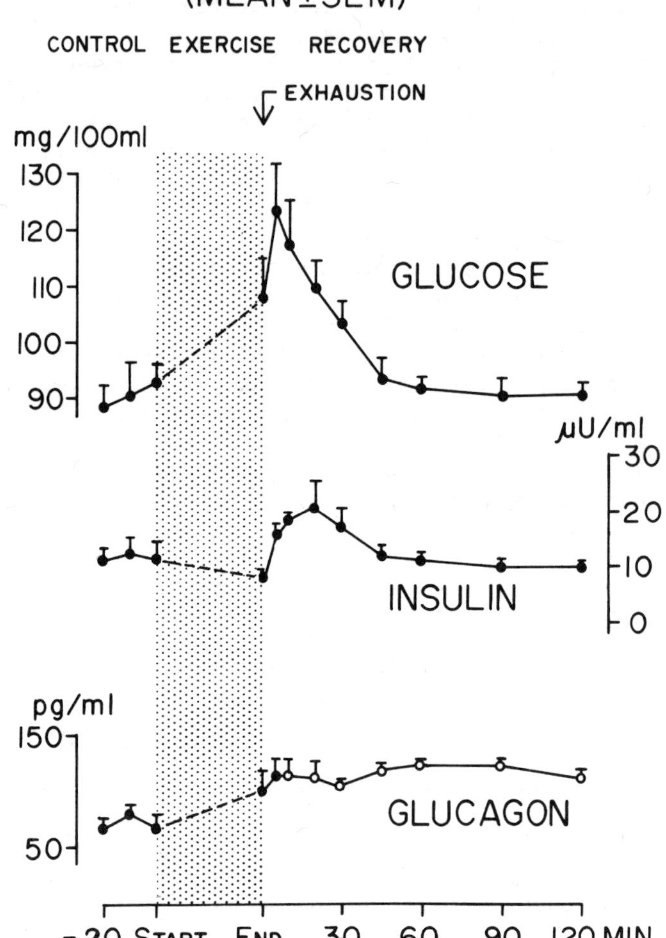

FIG. VI. The effect of strenuous treadmill exercise upon glucagon, insulin and glucose levels in a normal dog.

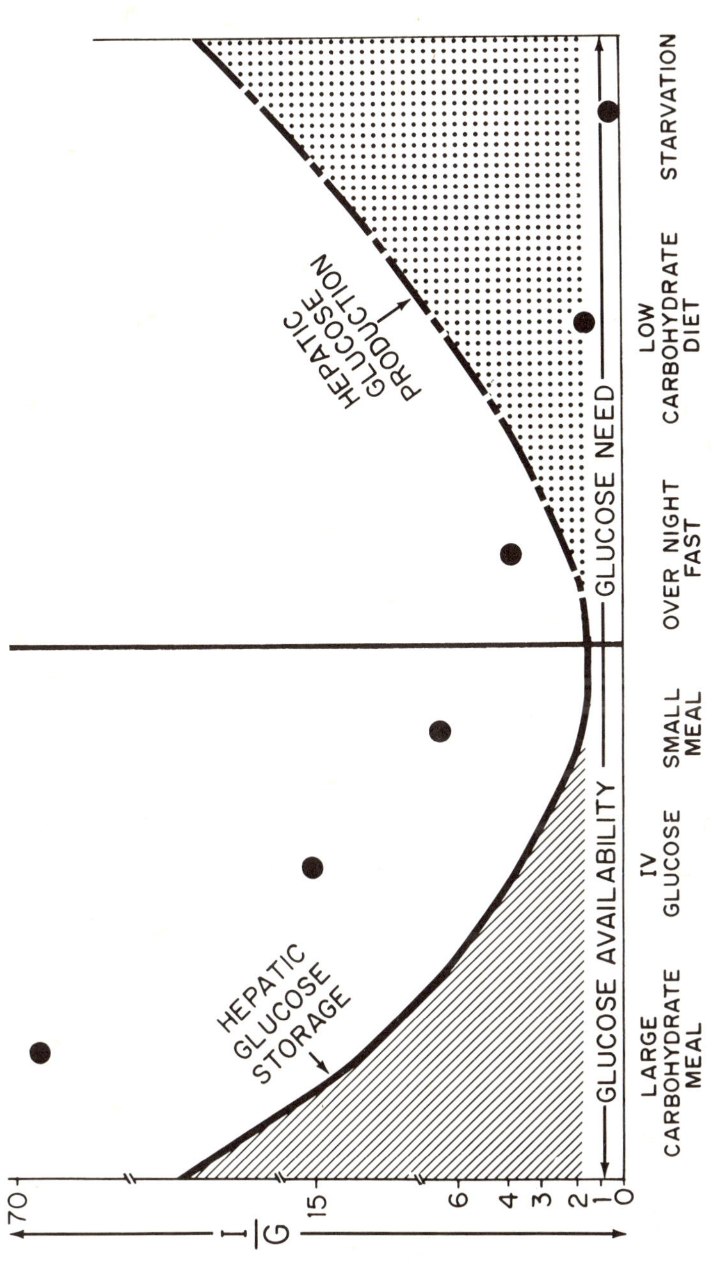

FIG. VII. The normal relationship between insulin/glucagon ratio (o) and fuel availability.

else to permit the glycogenesis?

DR. UNGER: That is an important point because in the case of exercise itself hyperglycemia is independent of the insulin.

In stress without muscular exercise, that is an important issue; no matter how high the glucose level goes, insulin will not respond, at least not fully. And if you look at patients who are admitted, let us say in vascular collapse, due to trauma, or burned patients receiving glucose I.V. and who have marked hyperglycemia, insulin levels are usually not high. The same low insulin glucagon ratio that prevails in severe exercise prevails also in starvation but is brought about by a reciprocal change in both hormones; a lowering of insulin and an increase in the glucagon. This bi-hormonal change is maintained during this critical period until the brain becomes adapted to the use of keto-acids.

The most important nutrient in the diet, in terms of long-term survival, is, of course, protein. Here again in the spectrum of glucose need, ranging from total starvation at one extreme to glu-cose abundance at the other, response of the alpha-beta cell couple of the insulin-glucagon ratio to a given amino acid load will vary tremendously. If, for example, one gives an amino acid load to a starving person, the insulin glucagon ratio will fall. This nega-tive insulin-glucagon ratio will predictably result in utilization of a high percentage of the incoming amino acids, not for protein synthesis, but for glyconeogenesis. The nitrogen, of course, is lost as urea. At the other extreme, the same amino acid load given to the same individuals during an intravenous glucose in-fusion or a high carbohydrate diet will result in a pronounced rise in insulin-glucagon ratio. This positive response to insulin-glucagon ratio will result in conservation of the amino acids for protein synthesis rather than for unnecessary gluconeogenesis. Well before the turn of the century it was known that glucose had a protein-sparing effect. We propose that the islet cells mediate this phenomenon.

The observation of Dudrick concerning the efficacy of hyper-alimentation may also reflect insulin-glucagon response to amino acids during glucose abundance (30). If you give intravenous amino acids without any glucose to a starving person, a fall in insulin-glucagon ratio will result. But, if you give them amino acids with glucose a rise in the insulin-glucagon ratio will occur. We emphasize the primacy of glucose in influencing the response of the islets of Langerhans to non-glucose nutrients. Here, with a normal glucose concentration, a response to a protein meal is one in which there is a small rise in insulin and a brisk rise in gluca-gon; by raising the glucose concentration, we abolish the glucagon response and enormously exaggerate the insulin response. This

should change the fate of the ingested amino acids. Fig. VIII
shows that if you put a large fat meal into the duodenum of a
conscious dog, insulin barely changes but glucagon goes up. Now
if the glucose concentration in the same dogs is raised by an I.V.
glucose infusion there is a huge response, over 300 micro-units
per ml., and instead of getting hyperglucagonemia, it is completely
suppressed.

DR. LEVINE: Roger, in the pancreas of the animal, the blood
in that animal "sees" a certain concentration of glucose, right?
That is, it responds to it. Now let us say it "sees" a concentration of 150 mg% and the beta cell shoots out a certain amount of
insulin. What makes it shoot out more insulin at the same glucose
level if there is fat in the gut?

DR. UNGER: I assume it is pancreozymin, or the gastric inhibi-
tory polypeptide (GIP); it is a gut hormone, that we know. It has
nothing to do with the chyle.

DR. LEVINE: But is it the kind of reaction which requires a
simultaneous rise in glucose? Otherwise it would not operate on the
beta cell. If it is an effect of the enteric hormone by itself,
then the giving of fat by itself should have done it; why does it
need the glucose?

DR. UNGER: To say that there is no insulin response whatever
is incorrect. There is a little response but it is small.

DR. LEVINE: But I do not mean that. What I mean is that there
was a response. The response with glucose alone would produce a
rise of 120 to 130 uU/ml. When the animal received the fat meal
into the duodenum accompanied by glucose administration, the rise
was 300 uU/ml. Is this because of a rise, or the presence of some
enteric factor? Can we say the enteric factor by itself is incon-
sequential?

DR. UNGER: Right. I want to turn now to a state in which the
                          alpha-beta cell couple is operating
The Effects   improperly, namely in stress hyper-
of Stress   glycemia, which I feel should be recog-
                          nized as a definite clinical entity. It
is undoubtedly the most common form of acute hyperglycemia seen in
an acute hospital. Stress hyperglycemia may be a device which permits the brain to maintain an adequate level of glucose delivery at
a time of reduction in cerebral blood flow. The only way adequate
glucose delivery can be maintained when cerebral blood flow drops,
is by raising arterial glucose concentration. Stress hyperglycemia
is a valuable response to shock.

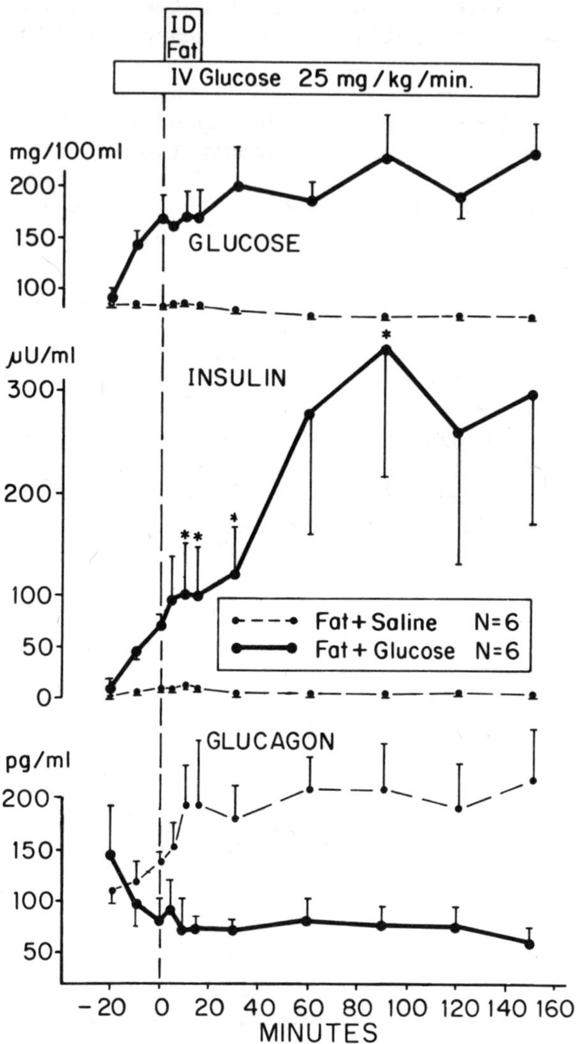

FIG VIII. The effect of exogenous hyperglycemia
upon the insulin and glucagon response to intraduodenal
fat in normal dogs.

Nevertheless in severe stress, even after glucose is provided
intravenously by the physician, the stressed islets appear incapable of relaxing; that is, the beta cells seem to respond normally
to hyperglycemia but the alpha cell cannot shoot off secretion of
glucagon. The presumably genetic abnormality known as diabetes,
affects the entire alpha-beta cell couple. As the beta cell seems
incapable of responding fully to the need for insulin secretion,
the alpha cell seems incapable of decreasing its secretion of glucagon even though glucagon may be unnecessary and may, in fact, be
detrimental to the organism. Thus far, several alpha cell abnormalities have been demonstrated in diabetes. During relative or
absolute hyperglucagonemia in the fasting state, or after a carbohydrate meal, or a glucose load, not only does glucagon fail to
decrease, but it often increases in a paradoxical fashion (see
Fig. IX).   And in the diabetic, irrespective of how much carbohydrate is ingested, protein stimulates a normal or supernormal
response of glucagon secretion. Finally, in diabetic ketoacidosis,
and in diabetic hyperosmolar coma, extreme hyperglucagonemia is
present. The mean fasting glucagon level in a large, non-diabetic
group is around 75 pg/ml, while in well-controlled diabetics it is
slightly but significantly higher. In uncontrolled diabetes, however, even though the blood glucose is extremely high, glucagon is
four or five times normal (see Fig. X). In the diabetic patient
failure to release enough insulin is coupled with an inability to
turn off glucagon. So again, there appears to be in this genetic
disease state a reciprocal defect in the alpha and beta cells.

DR. LEVINE: Now in the juvenile diabetic, a meal fails to
suppress glucagon secretion. What would be the result of adding
a little insulin with that meal?

DR. UNGER: It does not suppress the glucagon. If the relative concentration of insulin and glucagon is important in the
handling of a few nutrients, consider the plight of the juvenile
diabetic whose insulin level is constant, derived from whatever
he absorbs from a given dose that morning, when given an arginine
infusion, not only can he not increase his insulin, but his glucagon response is exaggerated. This insulin-glucagon ratio can only
go down in response to a protein meal. The fate of the amino acids
one would predict, would be different from the normal person. This
would be true even in a less severe diabetic person. It is note-
worthy that during arginine infusion in juvenile diabetics, the
glucose rise (in the fasting state) was about 65-75 mg % in 60
minutes (see Fig. XI). One wonders, then, as to the value of
glucagon suppression during a meal in such individuals. Could
one achieve any benefit by raising the insulin glucagon ratio -
that is by suppressing glucagon during this period of amino acid
influx - would this be beneficial? In any case, one would like to
think that, if this were possible, one could get a better compro-

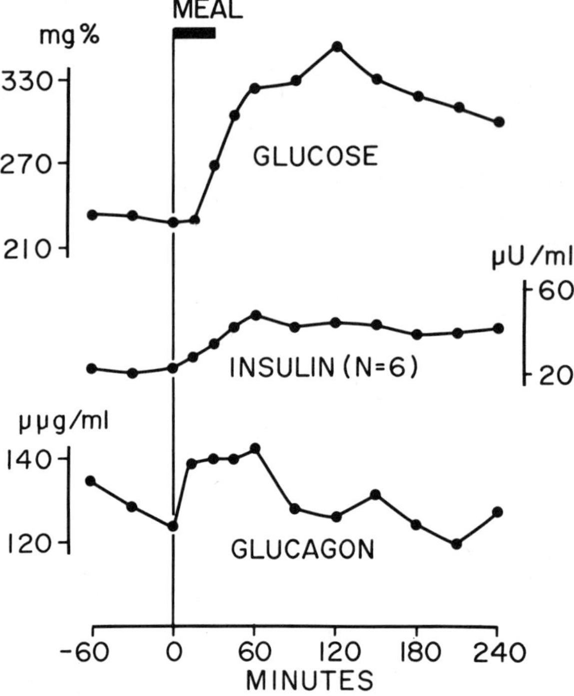

FIG. IX. The response of glucagon, insulin and
glucose to a large carbohydrate meal in 12 adult
onset type diabetics. The subnormal rise in insulin and the failure of glucagon to decline, despite the marked rise in plasma glucose, is in sharp
contrast to the normal response to such a meal.

mise between the dose of insulin required to minimize post-prandial
hyperglycemia, of course without inducing severe hypoglycemia
between meals.

Any severe illness in a non-diabetic is accompanied by hyperglucagonemia. Why in the diabetic patient does infection cause a
deterioration in diabetic control. Can hyperglucagonemia, which
is produced by infection by itself, even in non-diabetics, cause
the diabetic to go out of control? How important is glucagon in
all of this? Fig. XII shows experiments that were done with alloxan-
diabetic dogs. During one week they were observed on their usual
insulin dose, and as you can see, that under this usual insulin

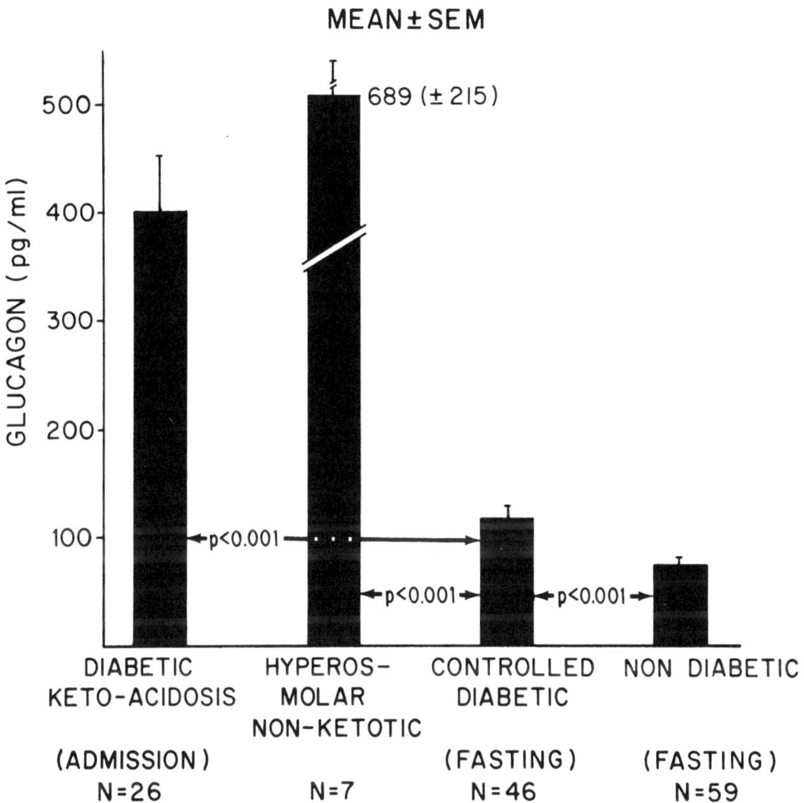

FIG. X. Plasma glucagon levels in uncontrolled and controlled diabetes mellitus as compared to non-diabetic subjects.

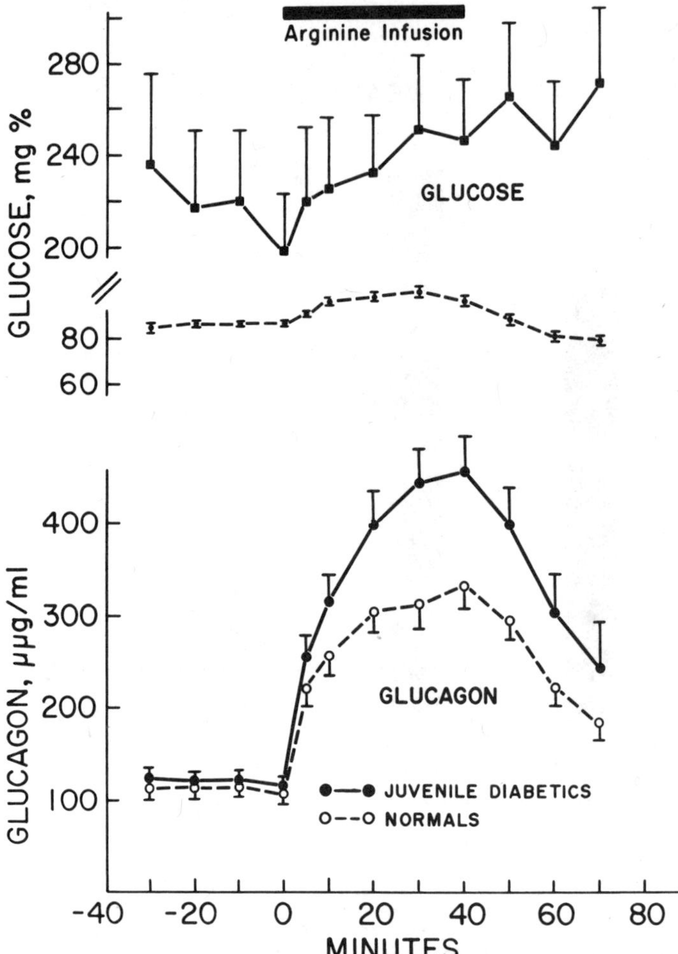

FIG. XI. The response of glucagon and glucose to arginine infusion in juvenile type diabetics compared to non-diabetic control subjects.

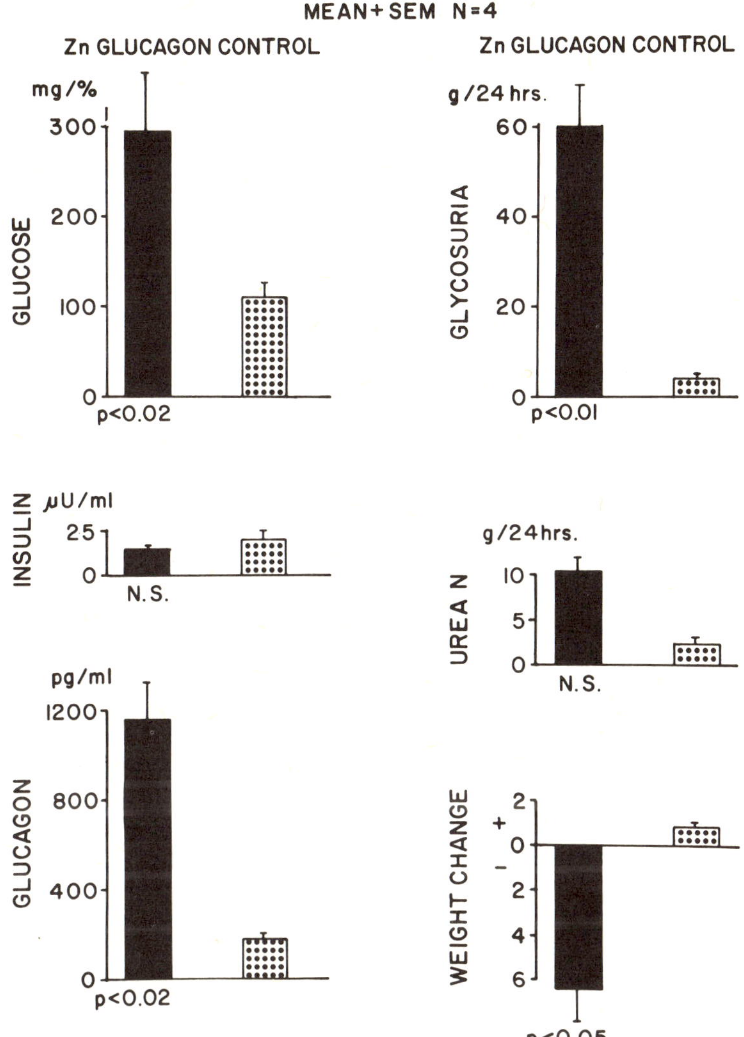

FIG. XII. The effect of exogenous hyperglucagonemia produced by daily injections of zinc glucagon upon blood glucose concentration, 24 hour excretion of glucose and urea, and body weight in a group of insulin-treated diabetic dogs. The closed bars represent the period of glucagon treatment and the stippled bars the control period. Despite the fact that insulin dosage and plasma insulin levels were the same, during the period of hyperglucagonemia, a marked increase in glycemia, glycosuria and urea was observed, together with a significant weight loss. These findings suggest that a fall in insulin glucagon ratio resulting from increased glucagonemia can cause a catabolic state.

dose they were rather well controlled; their fasting blood sugars averaged 100 mg %; they had very little glycosuria, a normal level of urea excretion, and therefore they maintained their weight. Then, for a similar week, with the same insulin dose, they were given zinc glucagon in an attempt to produce hyperglucagonemia of the magnitude which one would observe in a severe infectious condition. This hyperglucagonemia alone caused marked deterioration of diabetic control, with fasting glucose levels of over 300, marked increase in glycosuria (60 grams per day), a tripling of urea excretion and weight loss. In other words, a catabolic state was induced merely by adding glucagon.

Whatever produces an insulin deficiency results in glucagon secretion. Whether one uses alloxan or streptozotocin to damage the beta cells, or inhibits insulin secretion acutely with diazoxide or mannoheptulose, or neutralizes insulin with anti-insulin serum, there is an immediate rise in glucagon secretion. The one exception is somatostatin, and many of you heard Dr. Goodner report a remarkable and a very prompt reduction of insulin and glucagon when somatostatin is given (see Fig. XIII). Dr. Sakurai in our laboratory has studied this in six dogs. He noted that within one minute after the administration of somatostatin samples taken from the pancreatic vein show a reduction of 50% in the insulin and glucagon levels. Then within 2.5 minutes these substances approached unmeasurable levels in the assay. Yet with zero insulin there was no rise in glucose. In all other instances where the insulin levels reach zero, a rise in glucagon concentration as well as a rise in the level of glucose occur. The lack of glucagon is responsible for the lack of a glucose rise despite the zero insulin level, and if one adds glucagon prompt hyperglycemia occurs.

DR. WOLF: I don't mean to interrupt you Roger, but is there any evidence that the somatostatin in vivo actually circulates to the pancreas?

DR. UNGER: This is a pharmacological experiment and there is no knowledge on this as yet; we are just starting to do "dose-response" curves to see if one can get a pancreatic response at doses which would seem more realistic than the 200 microgram doses that we use for this. We are using it only as a pharmacological tool and not implying any physiological effect.

DR. WOLF: This is not something that you can detect in the blood?

DR. UNGER: There is as yet no assay for somatostatin. The administration of alanine causes a marked rise in glucagon and a

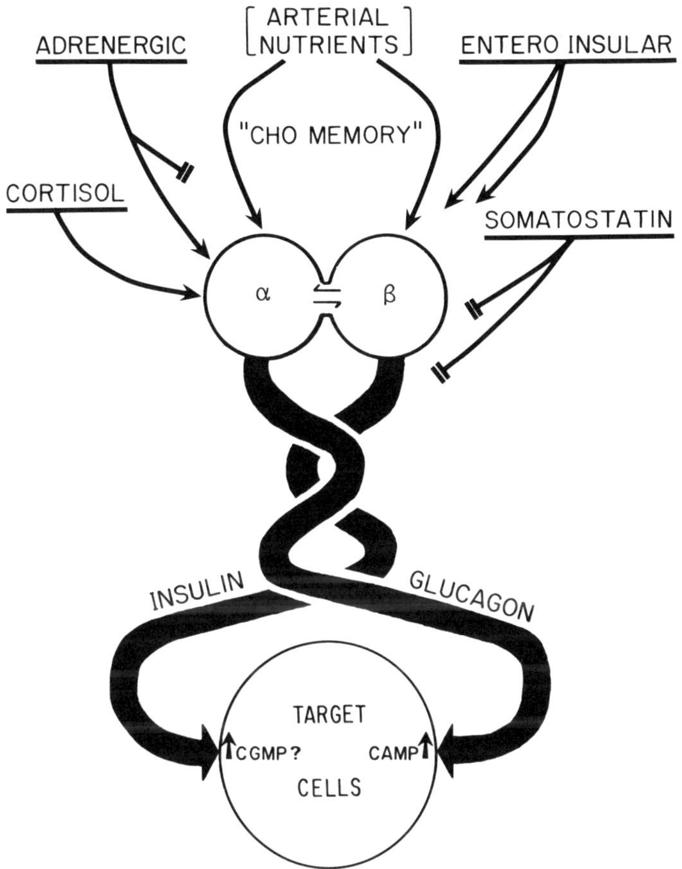

FIG. XIII. A schema depicting the controlling influences on the secretory output of the alpha-beta cell couple and the opposing effects of insulin and glucagon on common target tissues.

small rise in insulin and blood glucose rises about 15 mg %. However if somatostatin is given with the alanine infusion, there is no rise in either hormone and glucose concentration does not rise. We now have 10 dogs and the results are not impressive. These are long standing alloxan diabetic dogs, some of them more than two years on insulin. If they are taken off insulin as we do periodically, they get sick and have to be put back on. In these dogs, during an alanine infusion, without somatostatin, glucagon goes up, and the glucose goes up about 40 mg % during this brief exposure to alanine for some 15 minutes. In diabetic dogs on somatostatin, there is suppression of glucagon and there is no increase in glucagon during the alanine infusion, and the blood glucose at the time of peak hyperglycemia in the control group is about 60 mg % lower.

So these data would provide at least modest support for the hope that one could, by lowering the glucagon level in diabetics during influx of even a gluconeogenic substrate such as alanine, reduce glucose concentration.

DR. LEVINE: What happens to glucagon in a surgically totally depancreatized animal?

DR. UNGER: Dr. Orci has shown that in addition to the GLI producing cells in dogs and cats, there exist alpha cells in the gut which are indistinguishable from the alpha cells that normally occur in the pancreas and when the animal has recovered from the pancreatectomy, his response is the same as that of an alloxanized animal. Other workers found even higher levels of glucagon in the pancreatectomized dog than in the normal, but only in response to an amino acid such as arginine, and not when given insulin only. The source for this is the gut.

DR. LEVINE: Roger, were you able to use somatostatin in depancreatized animals that presumably had glucagon sources from the gut? Does it suppress it?

DR. UNGER: No, we have not done this yet in any depancreatized animals. We have studied it only in alloxanized diabetic dogs.

DR. ORCI: If you show a specimen of gut (the jejunum, for example) with alpha cells, to a cytologist he will not be able to distinguish whether these alpha cells are from the gut or from the pancreas. But this exists only in the dog and in the cat, and not in the rat.

DR. LEVINE: Lelio is a very nice guy and he can find cells wherever he seems to want to find them.

DR. ORCI: These are not the gastrin producing cells! But
this exists only in the cat and in the dog and the alpha cells are
the same as those found in the intact pancreas. The cytologist
cannot distinguish the location from whence they came.

DR. UNGER: Following a total pancreatectomy in some of these
animals the glucagon levels went to
zero when insulin was given; they were
responding in an exaggerated manner to
an amino acid infusion, in other words
The nitrogen sparing
effects of carbohydrates
they were acting just like alloxanized animals. We made discrim-
inatory assays of various parts of the gut looking for extra pancreatic glucagon. Finally this week we discovered a true glucagon
different from GLI but indistinguishable from pancreatic glucagon.

DR. LEVINE: You imply that the nitrogen-sparing action of
carbohydrate in depancreatized animals, or maybe better in normal
animals, is due to a combination of the suppression of glucagon and
the stimulation of insulin.

DR. UNGER: Right.

DR. LEVINE: Well, in the untreated depancreatized animals,
the infusion of carbohydrate is definitely nitrogen-sparing without the exhibition of insulin. Arthur Mirsky was really the one
who showed us that in the completely depancreatized animal who has
no insulin whatsoever, if glucose is infused, then you will get
very good nitrogen-sparing effects (87). Now I wonder what is
happening there, where there is not supposed to be any stimulation
of insulin or any suppression of glucagon. This is in the dog.

DR. WILLIAMS: And also, then you ran into more glucose utilization.

DR. LEVINE: Insulin suppresses nitrogen excretion in the
diabetic dog, and yet you showed that it does not suppress glucagon.
There is no doubt in a diabetic dog, a depancreatized dog, the
administration of insulin suppresses nitrogen excretion and yet
you show that glucagon does not go down!

DR. UNGER: Absolutely! Because you are raising the insulin-
glucagon ratio, you show that you can overcome the effects of
either one.

DR. LEVINE: I don't get it. How does this happen? Where's
the mechanism for this? Here you are, the glucagon is pushing toward gluconeogenesis. You are saying that by merely raising the
level of insulin, you are independently promoting protein-synthesis
and therefore are decreasing the nitrogen excretion.

DR. UNGER: I am saying that at any given level of glucagon,
you can give enough insulin to over-ride the effects of glucagon.

DR. LEVINE: O.K., that's fine, but that does not explain
the nitrogen-sparing effect of carbohydrate in the absence of either
hormone.

DR. UNGER: I would like to see that in a totally depancreatized animal or in a juvenile diabetic in whom there is no insulin.

DR. LEVINE: In a totally depancreatized animal, we've done
it; in a juvenile diabetic, I wouldn't dare do it.

DR. UNGER: I would like to see the hormone levels in your
experiments. We have had a great deal of difficulty in this work
to prove the total absence of hormone levels ...

DR. LEVINE: Well, hormone levels at the time we didn't have
and we didn't do them. But at that time we observed blood sugars
between 400-700 mg % with ketosis.

DR. UNGER: May I ask you how those experiments were done?
What were their fasting glucose?

DR. LEVINE: I don't remember the exact details.

DR. UNGER: Then how much nitrogen was spared?

DR. LEVINE: Oh, the nitrogen-sparing was something in the
order of 50-60% of that in the controlled group.

DR. UNGER: I cannot explain how in the absence of an increase
of insulin, you could have a nitrogen-sparing effect from glucose.
I can say if you volume expand a very sick dog (and presumably
these were very sick dogs) you will suppress glucagon just from
expanding volume. That is, if they were hypovolemic.

DR. LEVINE: These dogs were out of control for three days.
They were getting sick as this experiment was carried out over 8
to 10 hours, and we put these dogs back in their cages. I don't
remember all the details and I must go back to that work and review
the details.

DR. KNOWLES: Roger, if you infuse glucose as you did in many
of these experiments, you don't change the blood sugar levels, may
be. You don't increase your glucose levels much but you increase
your utilization and the net positive balance of glucose that has
to do with the liver being shut off. This would be my explanation
for your observation.

DR. LEVINE: But my question was that there was no chance of
evoking insulin in these animals and yet we got a nitrogen-sparing
action out of glucose that was administered. But these were experiments simply to find out whether you decreased or increased
nitrogen-sparing action by administration of glucose to a completely
depancreatized animal. They were designed to see what the urea
excretion was both before and after the administration of insulin.

DR. UNGER: If there were some insulin present, then the
administration of glucose would certainly have some nitrogen-sparing
effect.

DR. LEVINE: But, supposedly we start with zero insulin level
in depancreatized dogs.

DR. UNGER: Yes, supposedly — and that is the question!

DR. WILLIAMS: Roger, wouldn't you say that this generalization
is what accounts for quite a large number of observations that we
make with respect to changes in the rate of excretion of insulin
and glucagon; namely, situations that increase glucose oxidation
in the beta cell increase insulin secretion, whereas conditions
that decrease glucose oxidation in the alpha cell increase glucagon secretion.

DR. UNGER: Absolutely, I would agree with that.

DR. WILLIAMS: It seems to me that it explains these differences in observations.

DR. LEVINE: Does it mean that it has to be glucose oxidation
or is it a case of glucose attachment or reception?

DR. WILLIAMS: Well, you are going to consider anoxia, for
example, that will increase glucagon secretion without changing
the glucose while it decreases insulin secretion.

DR. LEVINE: How do you account for the effect of the insulin
secretory effect of non-utilizable sugars such as 3-alpha methyl
glucose?

DR. WILLIAMS: They are decreasing glucose oxidation in the
beta cell.

DR. LEVINE: Yes, and yet they decrease insulin secretion.

DR. UNGER: I don't know that Dr. Williams meant to imply that
was the mechanism of the effect and anything that interferes with
ATP production is a poison — abolishes the effects on the alpha
cell.

DR. LEVINE: Yes, but anything that interferes with ATP production can do many other things.

DR. WILLIAMS: I do not mean that this explains everything because I do not quite know where the amino acid effect fits in here.

DR. UNGER: Oh, I thought you were speaking in a teleologic
sense that when fuel is needed, there is a whole spectrum of such
changes.

DR. WILLIAMS: There have been a large number of studies on
this and it just seemed to me that it represents a common denomin-
ator of the dilemma.

DR. SPRITZ: Roger, could I ask you in this situation, how
does this relate to the etiology of the diabetic? Could you give
us some explanation?

DR. UNGER: Dr. Orci's Institute is called the Institute of
Histology and Embryology and I wish you would ask him this question.
As far as I know, the alpha and the beta cells arise from a common
origin and it is not unreasonable to think that a defect that is
inherited by the beta cell might also be shared by the alpha cell,
as it is expressed in "mirror image" form. Both seem to fail to
respond to a rising glucose concentration - the beta cell by failing
to increase its output of insulin, and the alpha cell by failing
to decrease it. The net result is what we are looking at.

DR. WOLF: Roger, there is just one final question: have you
measured the glucagon level in someone on the Atkins' diet?

DR. UNGER: I think we have demonstrated a very poor insulin
response to protein feeding on a carbohydrate-free diet and an
exaggerated glucagon response on the Atkins' diet.

DR. WOLF: Has this actually been done on obese humans?

DR. UNGER: That work was done on healthy medical students before the Atkins' diet, but the results would be substantially the
same.

DR. WOLF: Roger, can you tell us where gastrin would fit into
this picture? That is, the interaction between the alpha and beta
cells with the effects of gastrin.

DR. UNGER: I can't contribute much on that, but Dr. Orci can.

DR. ORCI: I cannot comment on this either. I would like only
to stress that, ultrastructurally, there are differences between
the gastrin-producing cell, found in the pylorus (43) and the
D-cells of the islets of Langerhans (presumed to produce gastrin)
(54). Braaten and colleagues reported a few days ago in Atlantic
City, that gastrin was assayable in pancreatic monolayer cultures
(12). If gastrin was to be produced in the pancreas, we strongly
believe that a cell type different from the D-cell, would be involved in its synthesis. This cell type is encountered only rarely
in our monolayer culture of endocrine pancreas (97).

DR. SPRITZ: I am curious about the role of the suppression
defect of glucagon as part of the primary etiology. Roger, do you
think you could make a case for those patients who exhibit hyperglycemia without any of the other etiologies, who continue to have
high secretions of insulin like we talked about today? Whether
insulin resistance is the whole story in those patients or can you
identify some independent glucagon non-suppressibility that expressed itself in the diabetic at a time when insulin secretion is
still normal or supernormal?

DR. UNGER: Whereas non-diabetics will respond to a carbohydrate meal with a fall in glucagon
as glucose rises, in presumably genetic
diabetes this is not the case. Even
if one creates a relatively normal
pattern of insulin, where it would

Failure of Glucose and
Insulin to suppress
Glucagon in Diabetes

reach its peak at 300 microunits per ml., there is no evidence of
hypoglycemia which might alter the response. In any case, in these
ten diabetic individuals, the glucagon concentration did not change
during a carbohydrate meal accompanied by exogenous insulin. Moreover, even if one infuses insulin and glucose and uses large doses
of insulin so as to raise the blood level to pharmacologic levels
and administers glucose to prevent hypoglycemia, one does not see
the type of glucagon suppression that occurs in the non-diabetic
with the same level of hyperglycemia with only endogenous levels
of insulin of only 30 to 45 microunits per ml. So 1500 microunits
per ml. did not produce prompt suppression of glucagon in the diabetics. However, it does become statistically significant at these
points, but hardly is as substantial as is the case in the normal.
Now we are repeating these experiments using much lower doses and
comparing the adult and juvenile type of diabetics. But at the
present time we do not have enough data to quantitate what seems
to be an insulin resistant glucose or hyporesponsiveness of the
alpha cell. In experimental diabetes one can promptly correct the
hyperglucagonemia of insulin deficiency with small amounts of insulin.

DR. CAHILL: If you took this same diabetic and got his blood glucose up to 100 to 150 range for a couple of days while saturating him with insulin, would you then improve the glucagon responsitivity?

DR. UNGER: I cannot answer that because we have not done that type of experiment. We have looked at a large number of diabetics some of whom were very well controlled. Those with fasting blood sugars of, say, under 110 had higher glucagon levels than those in the 150 to 200 mg % range. Whereas if they went out of control to the point of having symptoms then their glucagon went much higher so we cannot say that there was any relationship to the fasting glucose concentration.

DR. CAHILL: What is the glucose suppressibility of glucagon?

DR. UNGER: We have not looked at it beyond 180 minutes testing.

DR. SPRITZ: Are these all non-obese diabetics, and are they adult-onset diabetics?

DR. UNGER: Yes. They are all less than 20% over their normal body weight. I would like to show you the dramatic effect of insulin in restoring hyperglycemic responses of the alpha cell in experimental diabetes. In a normal dog there is a normal response when blood sugar rises. There is a rise in insulin and a reciprocal fall in glucagon. But the alloxan-diabetic dog is incapable of raising his insulin in response to an increased concentration of glucose (Fig. XIV). The glucagon level goes up with the hyperglycemia. But when you give insulin with the glucose the glucagon level will go down. And in the case of this dog with a glucagon level of 14,000 picograms per ml., even though his glucose level was very, very high, just enough insulin to raise his serum level 30 or 40 microunits caused a precipitous fall in glucagon.

Chronic alloxan-diabetic dogs also respond (see Fig. XV). Dogs that have been diabetic for two years respond the same as normal humans do when they are given a normal amount of insulin, whereas in the ten adult diabetics even pharmacological levels of insulin restored very little of the glucagon responsiveness to hyperglycemia. So, therefore, the question is whether there is some specific lesion, in which the alpha cell cannot respond to glucose irrespective of insulin concentration. Or at least, they cannot respond in a normal fashion.

DR. SPRITZ: It is interesting to note that those alpha cells are turned off by somatostatin.

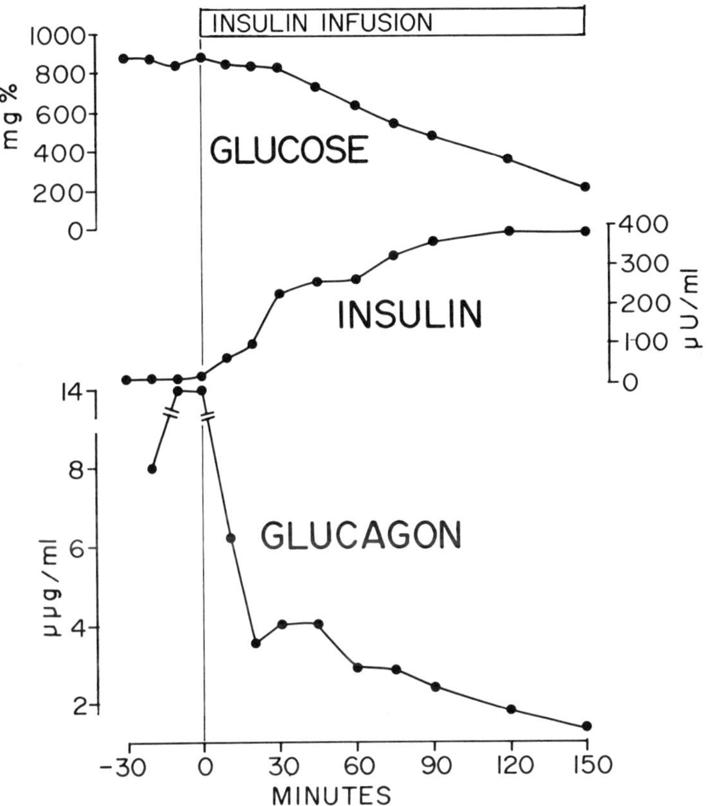

FIG. XIV. Plasma glucagon response to insulin in an alloxan-diabetic dog.

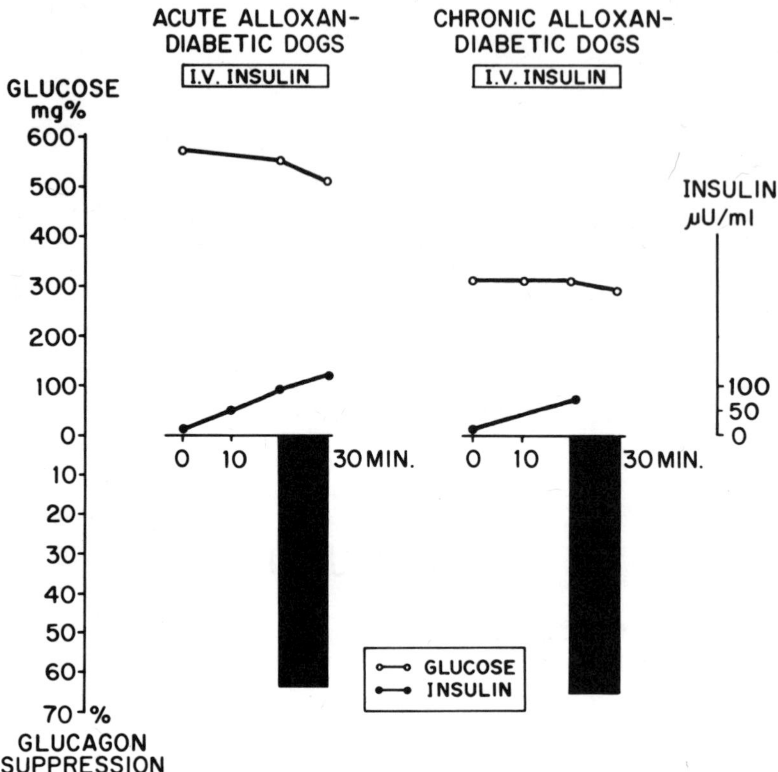

FIG. XV.   Comparison of alpha-cell suppressibility
(closed bars) during the infusion of insulin in
hyperglycemic dogs with alloxan-diabetes of short
and long duration.

DR. UNGER: Well, that is in experimental diabetes. It only
goes down to about 50%, you don't get complete suppression. You
still get a substantial reduction. I think that Dr. Forsham is
studying humans.

DR. SPRITZ: Roger, how do we fit this lack of suppression
of glucagon as associated with the etiology of diabetes?

DR. UNGER: I am beginning to think that it is very important.
In looking at some of the data of Vranic in his in vivo studies
and some of Lindquist's studies, it is relatively difficult to
overcome with insulin some of the effects of glucagon on the liver.
So that, if the liver is playing the major role, as some of us
believe, in regulation of glucose concentration, then glucagon
might be making a major contribution. I think it would be wise to

put forth a major effort to examine the effect of glucagon suppression more carefully than has heretofore been possible and see if this is, indeed, the case. The ideal, I think, would be this. Let us say we are controlling a juvenile diabetic with insulin (and this might have some application for the insulin pump with a glucose sensor), obviously we would want to limit post-prandial hyperglycemia and also to minimize hypoglycemia between meals. If we could get a suppression of glucagon when the individual eats his meal, I would suspect that we could maintain him with a normal level of insulin. The juvenile diabetic, if he eats a steak, cannot raise his insulin. There is an exaggerated glucagon rise so that, if the relative concentration of the two hormones is meaningful in terms of glucose homeostasis, that ratio can only go down in a catabolic direction. I just wonder if raising the insulin-glucagon ratio by dropping glucagon transiently, as with somatostatin, would not permit a level of insulin that would be much lower than what we now give to the diabetic. May be and may be not, but I think it is worth looking into.

DR. CAHILL: I would like to back that up completely. In addition the liver (when insulin is given peripherally) will always have a higher relative concentration of glucagon than insulin because the liver "sees" the pancreatic glucagon production in high concentration, but it only "sees" the peripheral <u>arterial insulin</u> concentration. Therefore, the diabetic is worse off on two factors. One is that he is endogenously hypoinsulinemic, and what insulin is given never reaches the same concentration as that which is reproduced in his own beta cells.

DR. LEVINE: Is there any work in which the depancreatized animal under non-anesthesia conditions is given an infusion of insulin to a certain degree of regulation and then is given glucagon after infusion, and is there a titration of one against the other?

DR. CAHILL: Yes. Cherrington, Vranic and colleagues have done this (22).

DR. LEVINE: Well, how much insulin was required?

DR. UNGER: There are some very interesting studies by two independent groups, one working in vitro at the Salk Institute (Dr. Leffert) at LaJolla, and the other is a surgeon, Dr. Price at P&S. And to make a long story short, their evidence shows that hepatic cell regeneration requires insulin and this is inhibited by too much glucagon. In Leffert's culture studies at a ratio of below 5 of insulin to glucagon he gets very little replication once the liver cells are in a quiescent phase. And then when he raises the ratio by increasing insulin, they begin to replicate again.

From this, one wonders whether cells with a glucagon receptor, other than the liver cells, might not be influenced similarly with respect to cell regeneration, namely conceivably the beta cells themselves. Whether in diabetes their replication is normal, or whether glucagon suppression might enhance this replication; perhaps there is some other factor that might enhance their beta cell mass also.

DR. WOLF: Do you know what the normal rate of replication is?

DR. UNGER: No, I do not think this has ever been studied either.

DR. CAHILL: The guess is that maybe it is like liver. In other words, once a year, i.e., one mitosis per year, which is a very slow rate and this is based on very circumstantial evidence. But it is a very slow process.

DR. WILLIAMS: I am impressed with patients who have had insulinoma for twenty years and yet do not have a myocardial infarction.

Insulin-Glucagon Relationships in Pancreatic Tumors

DR. LEVINE: Yes, that is true and obesity in general is an argument against this.

DR. WOLF: What happens to the patient with an insulinoma? Do you have any data on this?

DR. UNGER: There are good data but they have always been disappointingly flat: i.e., the glucagon response. Even with marked hypoglycemia, say around 20, you will never get much hyperglucagonemia. The reason for this, we think, is that in hypoglycemia which is caused by a high insulin, the alpha cell is deceived so that even at a low arterial concentration of glucose the high insulin permits penetration but to a degree which deceives the alpha cell, and this restricts an outpouring of glucagon. If, for example, you produce hypoglycemia in a dog by infusing insulin and by this means get the blood sugar down to, let us say, 30 mg %, the glucagon level will rise and after about 60 minutes it will then level off to slightly above normal. On the other hand, if you produced a blood sugar of 50 mg % by Phloridzin you will get a glucagon level of around 500.

DR. LEVINE: But, Roger, then that means that the alpha cell must sense something else than concentration. In other words, no matter how much insulin you have, to keep the sugar inside the cell into which insulin will push it, you are never going to go higher than the outside. The signal cannot be the concentration.

DR. UNGER: The signal is a function of the concentration of
both insulin and glucose and if that is the signal you could get
entry of glucose into the alpha cell.

DR. LEVINE: The signal cannot be the factor of concentration.

DR. UNGER: Let us take an example.   Let us say with 10 microunits of insulin, and if you produced hypoglycemia due to Phloridzin
then your insulin concentration will be about 2, 3 or 4 microunits
per ml. - way way down.

DR. LEVINE: You just cannot multiply two figures because if
you think that insulin makes the sugar go across, and into the
membrane ...

DR. UNGER: If penetration of glucose is dose related to
insulin, at least in a certain range ...

DR. LEVINE: Yes, but penetration may be dose related, but if
the alpha cell uses the concentration of glucose as a signal, then
it cannot go higher.

DR. UNGER: There is another explanation too, which I was
coming to, and that was what Samols was doing.   Namely, that insulin feeds back directly on the alpha cell and the output of
glucagon.   And if indeed you give a phloridzinized dog insulin,
you will lower his glucagon, but still that can be explained either
by the penetration index idea or the direct negative feed-back
effect.   The only way to test this is in vitro and we are trying to
do that now, and of course as yet we do not have the answer.

DR. CAHILL: Have you ever done this in Type I glycogenosis
(Von Gierke's Disease)?   We have two of them now where their blood
glucoses came down and we could not see any increase in glucagon.

DR. UNGER: And with relatively low insulins?

DR. CAHILL: Oh, undetectable -- but that may suggest some
chronic adaptation of the alpha cells to low glucose.

DR. UNGER: Well yes, like alcoholic hypoglycemics that are
supposed to give you high glucagon.

DR. CAHILL: Yes, but note also that with one tumor, a mesothe-
lioma, we could not get any increase in glucagon even with hypoglycemia.

DR. UNGER: They are much more chronic than in the animal and
when I said "chronic with phloridzin" I meant three or four days.

DR. WILLIAMS: The way you describe this thing fits when you have the normal regulation mechanism taking place, because we have several cases of insulinoma.

DR. WOLF: You mean islet tumors.

DR. WILLIAMS: Yes, islet tumors, where the amount of glucagon secreted is tremendous; there has been marked variation in this among patients with islet cell tumors. As with adenomas in general there is a loss of normal control mechanisms. There are quite a number of these people who, under certain conditions, not only secrete a tremendous quantity of insulin and glucagon, but also gastrin. This signifies a lack of differentiation in these tumor cells.

DR. CAHILL: There are several tumors now that are both glucagon and insulin producers.

DR. ORCI: Recently in Boston we received a tumor that is possibly an insulinoma. It was a multiple tumor and each one of the segments of the tumor contained a different type of cell. We were surprised to see this because, previously, we had seen tumors that were either those of the alpha cell or the beta cell, not different tumors of different cells in the same case; that is they were two different nodules with two different kinds of cells.

DR. CAHILL: Pearse thinks now that the carcinoid tumor produces bradykinin as well as serotonin and is a double cell tumor, one cell making serotonin and the other cell being a malignancy of a different type (108).

DR. SPRITZ: Supposing we take a case of an adult diabetic who did not suppress his glucagon output with insulin and glucose administration. I wonder whether you have ever done that experiment with glucose and tolbutamide rather than with insulin, on the assumption that tolbutamide would produce a high insulin level at the junction of the alpha and beta cells.

DR. CAHILL: Arginine or alanine stimulation might provide an answer also.

DR. UNGER: Samols has done some experiments with the sulfonylureas and so have we. Samols reports suppression of glucagon but no one has been able to confirm this (123). He carried out these experiments in ducks. It is the way to get the highest level of insulin in association with high blood sugars in the area of the alpha cell, as compared to the insulin infusion.

DR. CAHILL: Growth hormone levels are varied in diabetes.
The better you treat the diabetes, how-
Growth Hormone   ever, the further the growth hormone
level comes down.   And you find if you
treat the diabetes perfectly, there may be no excess growth hormone.
Growth hormone is normally secreted on the down side of a glucose
tolerance curve.   In diabetes this elevation of growth hormone in
response to a falling glucose level is exaggerated.

DR. LEVINE: What do we know about the biological significance
of these levels of growth hormone?

DR. CAHILL: We know there is absolutely no metabolic change
at the time of an acute spurt of growth hormone as evidenced by free
fatty acids, glucose resistance, etc. etc.   Most people are beginning to think that all of the metabolic effects of growth hormone
are expressed through somatomedin, and this is a long-delayed
effect.   That is why hypopituitary patients on just two injections
a week of 5 mg. of growth hormone, which has a half-life of just
30/40 minutes, grow.   Their insulin levels return to normal and
thus show the mild insulin resistance that all of us have because
of our own growth hormone; hypopituitary patients often will have
half the insulin levels of normals, because they have lost this
little bit of insulin resistance and do not have to overcome as
much growth hormone, but that all seems to be due to somatomedin.

DR. LEVINE: Hasn't it been shown that somatomedin has a pro-
liferating effect on the beta cells?

DR. CAHILL: I don't know.   We haven't done that.   We have
tried it in culture and I don't know of anyone who has added somatomedin in vitro.   But there is no question but that fibroblasts can
be maintained in vitro with somatomedin in certain cultures.   But
certain cultures require insulin, chicken fibroblast for example;
without insulin they will not grow.   Another point is that somatomedin is able to completely replace insulin, and also Nonsuppres-
sible Insulin-Like Activity, and these all have to be sorted out.

DR. SPRITZ: In the population with diabetes that we have
talked about, with very little vascular disease, are there studies
with reference to their growth hormone compared to other populations
such as Pima Indians, and so forth?

DR. CAHILL: Oh, the sexual ateliotic dwarfs have no detectable
amount.

DR. LEVINE: And the pygmy and Navajo populations with hyperglycemia and no vascular disease have a high growth hormone level
but it is not working in them.

DR. KNOWLES: It appears that there is a decrease in liver
clearance of growth hormone - as measured by the decay rate.

DR. WOLF: Dr. Cahill, you have pointed out the increase
in growth hormone in response to stimuli such as hypoglycemia;
therefore, do we have evidence in diabetes of increased amount of
growth hormone during deep sleep?

DR. CAHILL: Well, I don't know of any studies on sleep but
during the day normal subjects show a rise in growth hormone after
a meal as well as during emotional stress, exercise and other
daily activities. Children peak more frequently throughout the
day. Diabetics will also peak more frequently during the day.

If we could measure the mediator, somatomedin, with a good
antibody we might be able to tell what the integrated response of
somatomedin is to these peaks of growth hormone. All it takes is
one peak every two or three days in order to get normal growth
even in a hypopituitary patient.

The only way you can assay somatomedin is by sulfate incorporation into cartilage, or else tritiated thymidine and its incorporation into cartilage. In other words, you are really just measuring its end organ biophysiology. If somatomedin predisposes in
some way to the development of microvascular lesions, a trial of
therapy with depot somatostatin would be appropriate or some other
mechanism whereby we could inhibit growth hormone release, or by
neuro-adrenergics (such as dopamine and other agents that you could
use to alter hypothalamic-pituitary relationships). First, however,
we need to be able to follow somatomedin levels to get pure human
somatostatin in order to titrate and thus know whether we are doing
any good or not.

DR. CAHILL: Somatostatin will suppress growth hormone. In
fact, that is where it got its name - the suppression of somato-
tropin.

DR. KNOWLES: In our own studies we have higher growth hormone
levels in the retinopathy population. And in these patients, after
a meal, they do run a couple of nanograms higher than normal people
in both the girls and in the men. And these were the same values
that Floyd and Fajans got in Ann Arbor (67). But the reason for
this is what intrigues me and I don't know how accurate it is. The
studies have been done with labeled human growth hormone and it is
used in this form by all working with it.

In addition to that, we measured all the other pituitary factors
and particularly prolactins and found that they were pretty much
within our normal range in the juvenile diabetic males. In the

women they were about 3 or 4 nanograms higher and in patients with
diabetic nephropathy were about 7 nanograms higher. And LH and
FSH in the males were at the normal level. And the same with TSH.
I could not determine any gross abnormality in retinopathy because
they were about the same as in the normal, so therefore it was
difficult to attribute the retinopathy to a pituitary defect, ex-
cepting the 2 nanogram rise in growth hormone for both the girls and
the boys.

DR. LEVINE: Some people contend that microangiopathy and growth
hormone are related although that evidence is very poor. In a
group of dogs, following growth hormone and alloxanization, Bloodworth observed changes closely resembling the retinal changes in
men (9). There are pathologists who will not agree that the retinal changes in those animals and in some alloxanized rats, are
the same as the retinal changes found spontaneously in human diabetes.

DR. WOLF: Has it been possible to observe microvascular changes
in animals following alloxan or pancreatectomy without the addition
of growth hormone or anything else?

DR. LEVINE: Some people would contend "yes" but other people
will say that the pathology of those lesions is not the same as in
the kidney; for example, is not the same as that seen in diabetes
in man; the kidney lesion tends to resemble more what can be produced with cortisone in the normal, the so-called exudative lesion
rather than true nodular glomerulosclerosis.

DR. WILLIAMS: Essentially every hormone exerts some effect on
the status of diabetes. It has long been known that permanent
diabetes could be produced under certain conditions by the administration of large amounts of growth hormone, glucosteroids, or
glucagon, and that less insulin is required for the control of diabetes in the absence of growth hormone, glucosteroids, glucagon or
catecholamines. In juvenile diabetics plasma growth hormone levels
are hypernormal and fluctuate much more throughout the day than
in nondiabetics (55). Somatostatin has been shown not only to
inhibit secretion of growth hormone (14), but also of glucagon
and insulin in baboon, dog and rat (68, 120) and in man (1).
It decreases the rate of glucose utilization in man. Perfusion of
rat pancreas with somatostatin inhibits glucagon and insulin secretion (62). Incubation of somatostatin with isolated rat
islets does not inhibit insulin secretion. Infusion of somatostatin
in baboons causes hypoglycemia, presumably as a result of inhibition of glucagon or growth hormone secretion (68,120). Glucagon
exerts a marked stimulating effect on insulin secretion, and
affects in many ways its net action (74).

DR. LEVINE: Given adequate amino acids by way of protein in-
gestion the hypophysectomized and
Hormones and   pancreatectomized animal is quite cap-
Gluconeogenesis   able of gluconeogenesis although he
cannot mobilize his endogenous amino
acids for this purpose.   And therefore the substrate effect directly,
or by a metabolic flow, is performing the required metabolic steps.
Perhaps we place too much stress on the hormones as being responsible for, and directing, the whole situation.

DR. WILLIAMS: Well, such an animal would have a marked deficiency in glucosteroids because of the hypophysectomy and there
are reports that in the absence of glucosteroids, you would have a
very significant impairment of gluconeogenesis.

DR. LEVINE: Glucagon by itself cannot mobilize the amino
acid, but all you need to do is to give protein!

DR. CAHILL: The maximum capacity for gluconeogenesis in the
liver of the adrenalectomized animal is down, but there's still
enough reserve there that if you give it the load of protein by
feeding, it will maintain normal homeostasis.

DR. WILLIAMS: Many investigators have shown that substrate
supply is a major factor controlling gluconeogenesis, and liver
from rats fed a high protein diet when perfused with alanine or
pyruvate has more gluconeogenesis than does liver from normal fed
rats (32).

DR. LEVINE: It is true that if you tax the capacity of that
liver it will show a lesser capacity for gluconeogenesis in the
higher range but the basic biochemical mechanisms are present in
the absence of hormones or in the presence of very low hormone
levels.

DR. CAHILL: The diabetic liver is always poised more toward
glycogen breakdown and gluconeogenesis for a given concentration
of glucose that is circulating in the body.   So you are always
going to have a greater turnover.   Do you follow my logic?

DR. KNOWLES: George, has anybody measured the concentration
of exogenous insulin in the portal vein?

DR. CAHILL: Yes, in dogs a suppression of endogenous insulin
resulted and the portal concentration approached that of the peripheral circulation.   That is why I think that the ketone production
seen in hypoglycemic reactions in a diabetic or in hypoglycemia is
a function sometimes, of lowered insulin production in the pancreatic circuit of those people.   You can get a situation where

you can infuse insulin and lower blood glucose and lower amino acids so that the liver is really "seeing" less insulin than it did before you even started the reaction by endogenous suppression, by lowering substrate.

DR. UNGER: We see such an effect clinically, in those recovering from ketoacidosis where the phase of ketone production continues despite adequate concentrations of insulin and glucose. The phenomenon is probably explained by the fact that liver enzymes are slow in responding.

Chapter IV - STRUCTURAL ASPECTS OF ISLET CELL MEMBRANES

DR. ORCI: Despite a growing body of data on islet cell structure and function in spontaneous and experimental diabetes (100, 101
113, 114, 115), the basic lesion(s) responsible for endocrine pancreatic dysfunction in this disease remain(s) to be unraveled. Although
membrane systems are known to be of major importance in the control
of cellular activities, no information is so far available concerning the possible role of the membranes as a crucial factor in the
impairment of islet function in diabetes mellitus. In this presentation, attention is paid to some structural aspects of such membranes
in normal and diabetic animals. One of the most useful techniques
in the morphological study of membranes is the freeze-fracture technique (88, 132), which exposes large areas of the inside of membranes
in three-dimensional view (Figs. XVI and XVII provide a comparison
of conventional and freeze-fracturing techniques) and reveals individual components of these membranes down to a macromolecular size,
namely 20 to 30 angstroms. With this technique, the interior of
the membranes (middle of the bilayer) is exposed (13, 109), and
appears structurally differentiated into smooth areas interrupted
by particles 60 to 180 angstrom in diameter (Fig. XVIII). It is now
accepted that the smooth areas represent the membrane phospholipids
whereas the particles constitute at least in part, the morphological
counterparts of proteins (26, 34, 86, 124, 139). Together, proteins
and phospholipids are the building blocks of the membrane. Membranes
rich in proteins, thus functionally complex, contain numerous particles.

For studying the membrane of islet cells, we had first to find
a way of distinguishing A from B cells in freeze-fracture replicas.
Indeed, the usual criteria used in thin-sectioned material, for
example the electron-density of the granule core, and its distance
from the limiting membrane, cannot be used in a freeze-fracture
preparation, which being a replica of a frozen surface, gives no
indication concerning the electron-density of the tissue itself.
Previous attempts to differentiate A and B cells were based on
such crude and indirect evidence as the topographic location of
the cells within the islet (94), the B cells being situated at
least in some animal species, in the center of the islet (42, 94).

The animal chosen for the study of spontaneous diabetes, the
Chinese hamster, offers however a new and very secure morphological
criterion for identifying A cells in freeze-fracture. In this animal species A cells contain bundles of cytoplasmic fibrils in the
paranuclear region which are clearly identifiable in freeze-fracture
replicas (Fig. XVIV). Such bundles are virtually absent in the
B cells. Being able to distinguish A and B cells unequivocally,

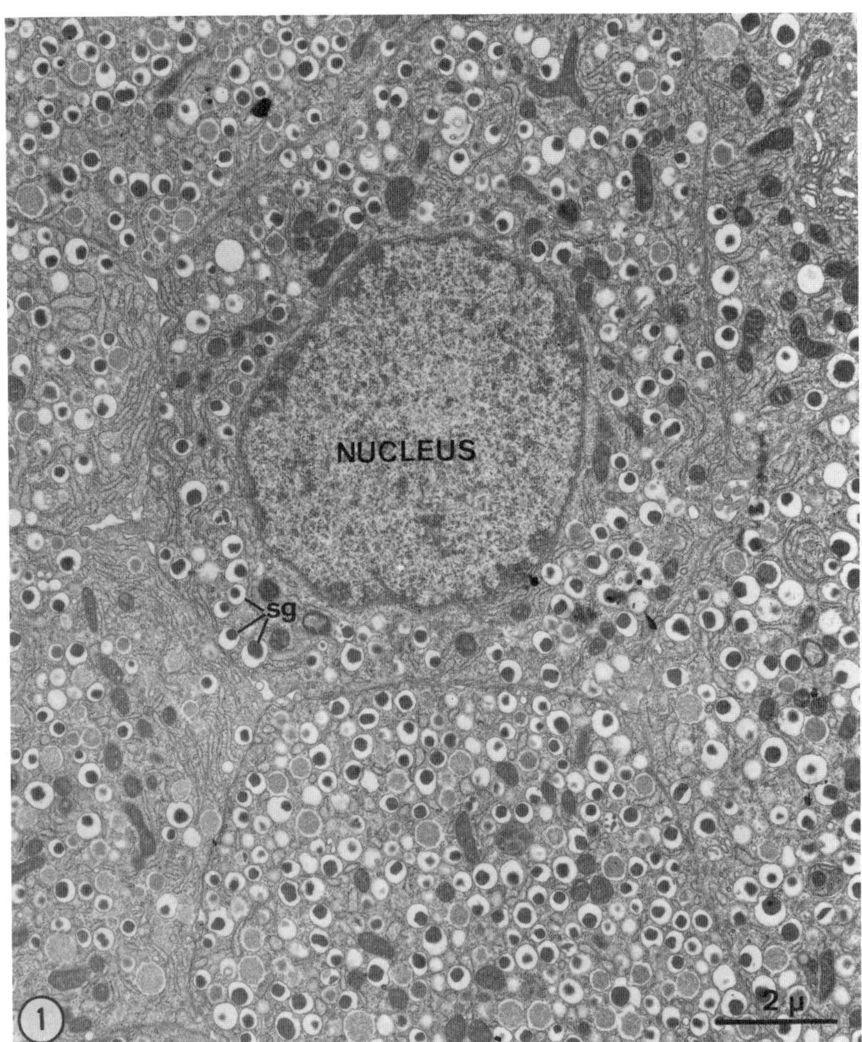

FIG. XVI. Rat islet. Thin section. The field shows several B-cells in which the most conspicuous organelles are the specific secretory granule (sg). The cell membranes are seen as faint dark lines.

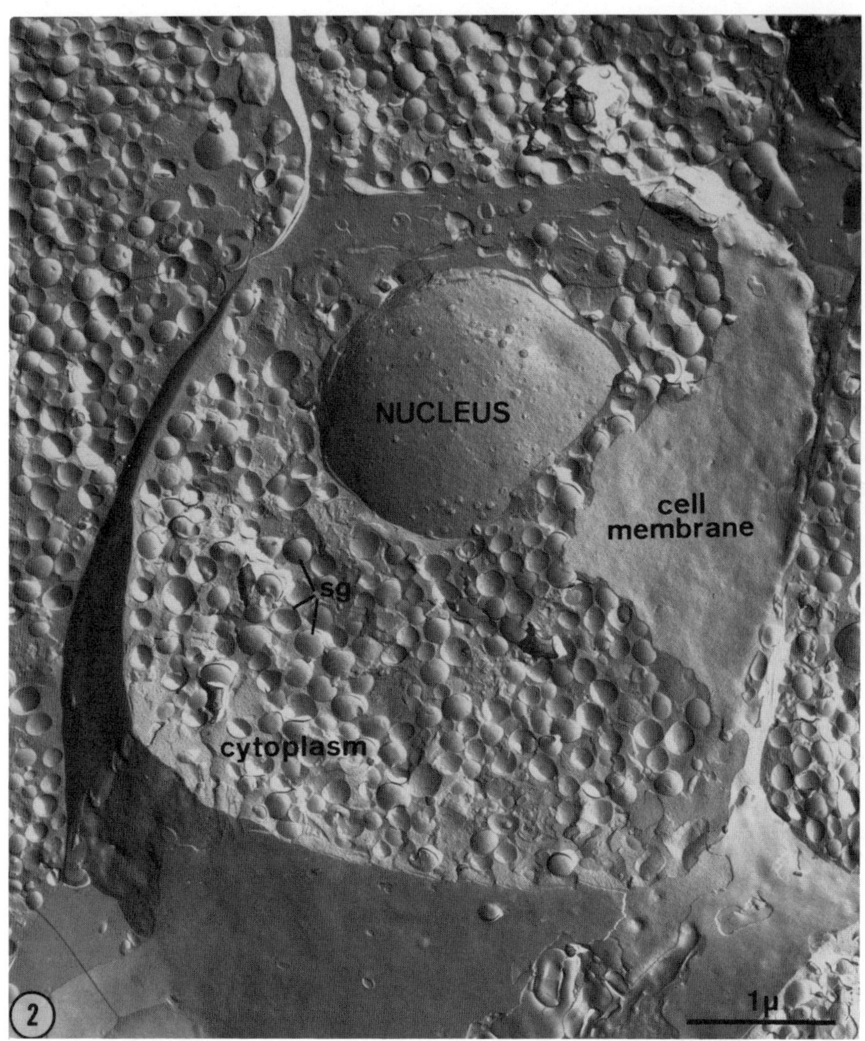

FIG. XVII. Rat islet. Freeze-fracture. In this
replica, both cytoplasmic and membrane fractures
can be seen. The cell membrane is largely exposed,
as is the membrane of the nuclear envelope. Within the cytoplasm, numerous globular elements represent the membrane of the secretory granules (sg).

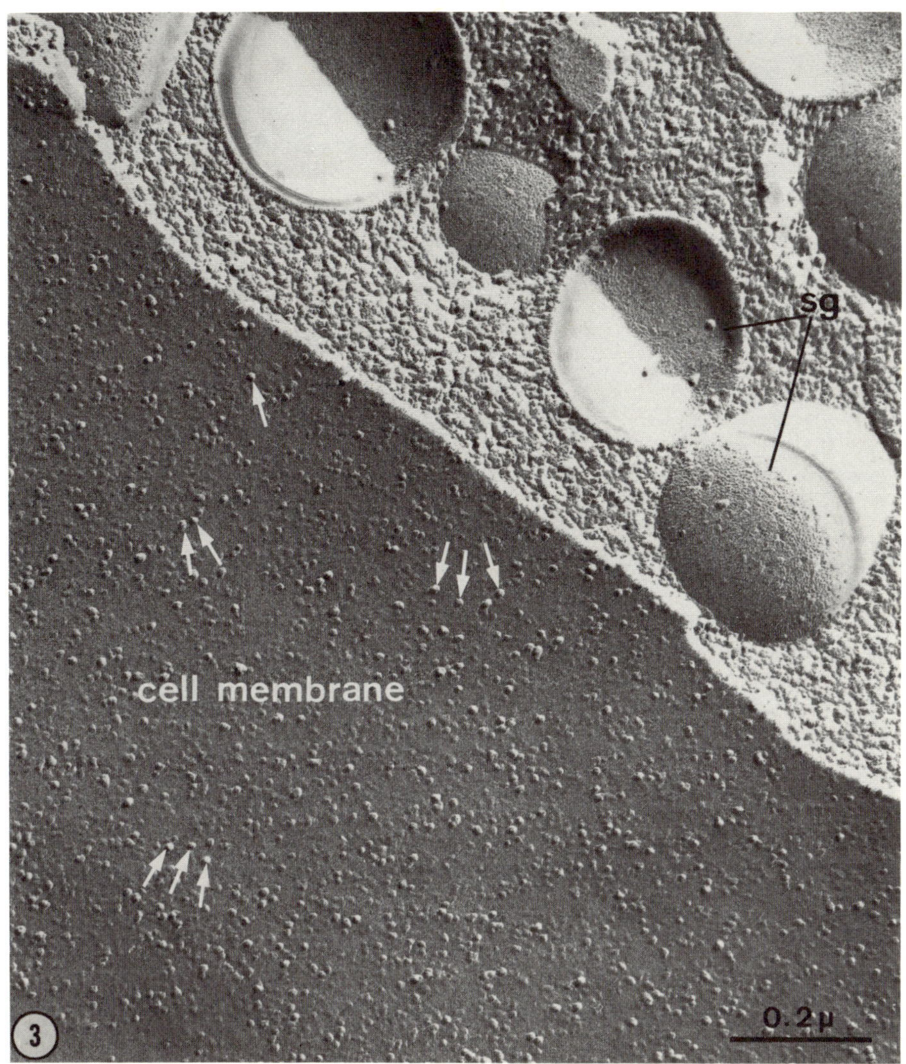

FIG. XVIII.   B-cell of normoglycemic Chinese hamster.
Freeze-fracture.   The inside of the cell membrane is
seen here at high magnification.   It is composed of
smooth areas (predominantly lipid) interrupted by random particles (arrows) (predominantly proteins).
sg = membrane faces limiting the secretory granules.
It is now widely accepted that the number and distribution
of intramembranous particles are related to functional
activity of biological membranes.

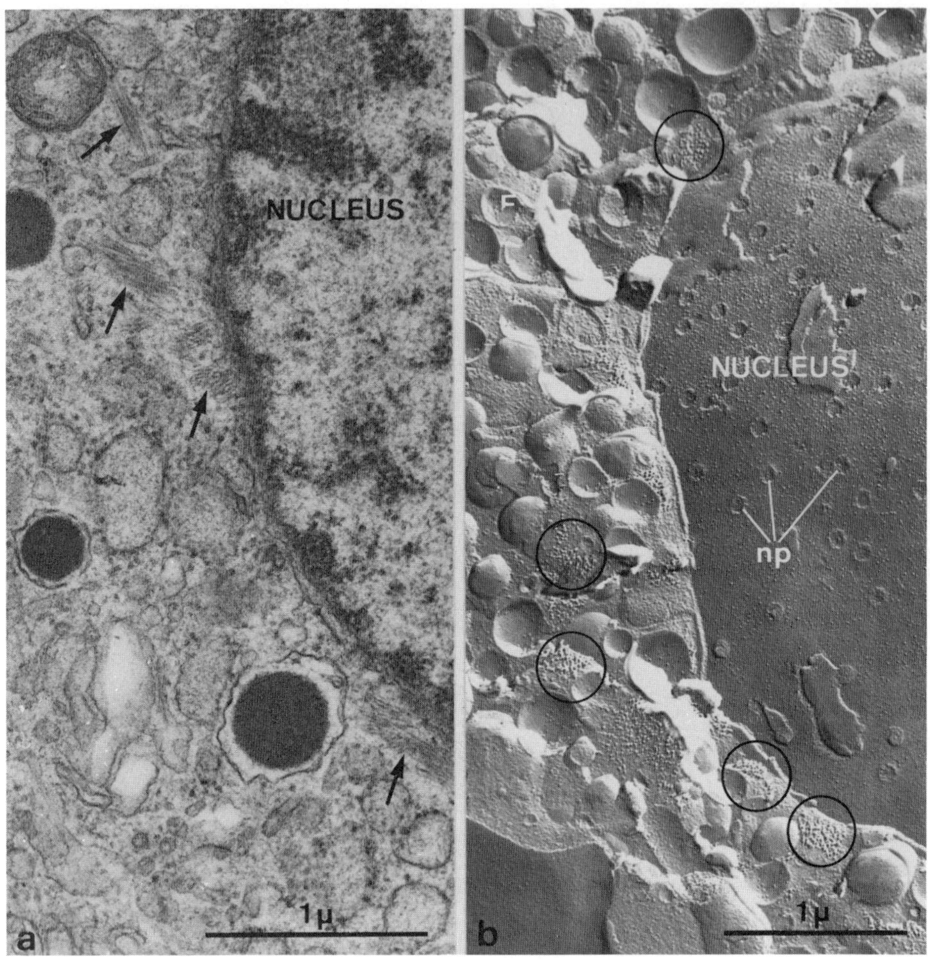

FIG. XIX.   A-cells of normoglycemic Chinese hamster.
Thin section (a) and freeze-fracture (b).   Bundles of
coarse filaments (tono-filaments; arrows in (a) and
encircled in (b)) are visible in perinuclear regions.
Such bundles of filaments are virtually absent in B-
and D-cells.   Moreover, D-cells are easily distinguish-
able from both A- and B-cells in freeze-fracture, since
their secretory granules are characteristically small
and polymorphous.   Nuclear pores (np) are clearly
visible in the membrane of the nuclear envelope.

we first turned our attention to the architecture of nuclear en-
velopes in both cell types. This problem was investigated since
we know that nucleo-cytoplasmic exchanges probably occur through
the nuclear pores and that such exchanges are instrumental in the
control of many cytoplasmic activities, for example cytoplasmic
syntheses (for review, see ref. 40). Fig. XX illustrates the results obtained by measuring the number of nuclear pores per square
micron of nuclear envelope for A and B cells. For each cell type,
we have compared the data obtained in 5 pairs of control Chinese
hamsters, 5 pairs of non-ketotic diabetic animals, and 5 pairs of
ketotic hamsters.**

     For the A cells, the density of nuclear pores was significantly
                              higher in ketotic diabetic animals than
Nuclear pores and   in control animals, the non-ketotic
membrane particles   diabetic animals occupying an intermed-
                             iate position. A comparable pattern
was found for the B cells, the major difference being seen between
control and diabetic animals, whether these latter were ketotic or
non-ketotic. The increase in the number of nuclear pores observed
in A cells during the course of diabetes mellitus could reflect
more nucleo-cytoplasmic exchange which in turn could be indicative
of an increase in the biosynthetic activity of glucagon-secreting
cells. If true, this interpretation supports the view that a
relative increase in glucagon production contributes to the development of the hyperglycemic syndrome in the Chinese hamster. Like-
wise, the increase in the number of nuclear pores observed in B
cells of diabetic Chinese hamsters could also indicate an increased
biosynthetic activity of the insulin-producing cells and, as such,
is consistent with previous claims that the relative insulin deficiency seen in these animals cannot be ascribed to a primary defect in the synthesis of the hormone (82). A second parameter
studied in A and B cells was the number of particles present in
the plasma membrane of each cell type. The density and the pattern
of distribution of these particles were studied in both normal and
diabetic animals. The numerical density of particles in the plasma
membranes of A and B cells is shown in Fig. XXI. For the B cells,
a progressive and highly significant fall in the density of the

---

**   The Chinese hamsters were obtained from a colony maintained at
     the Upjohn Company, Kalamazoo, Michigan. Mean plasma glucose
     levels at the time of sacrifice averaged 107 $\pm$ 4, 256 $\pm$ 23, and
     320$\pm$ 13 mg / 100 ml., in the aglycosuric, glycosuric and both
     glycosuric and ketonuric animals, respectively. (See L. Orci,
     M. Amberdt, F. Malaisse-Lagae, A. Perrelet, W. E. Dulin, G. C.
     Gerritsen, W. J. Malaisse, A. E. Renold. Diabetologia 10: 529-
     539, 1974). We thank Drs. W. E. Dulin and G. C. Gerritsen of
     the Upjohn Company for supply and selection of these animals.

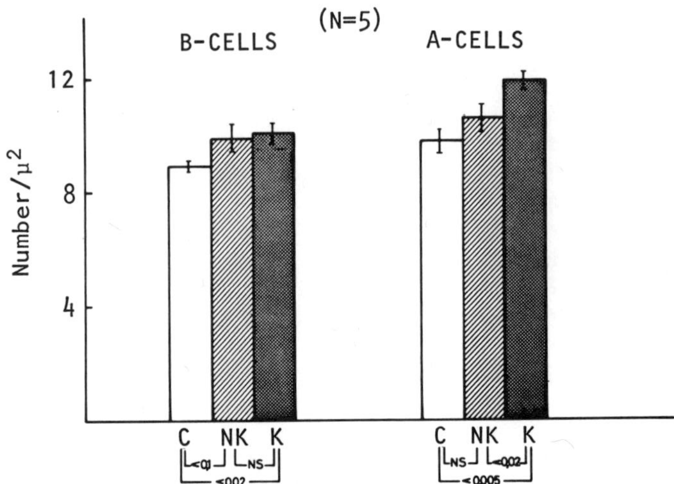

FIG. XX. Number ($\pm$ SEM) of nuclear pores per μ^2 of nuclear envelope in B- and A-cells of control (C), diabetic (NK) and ketotic (K) Chinese hamsters. Also indicated is the statistical significance of the observed differences (NS = not significant).

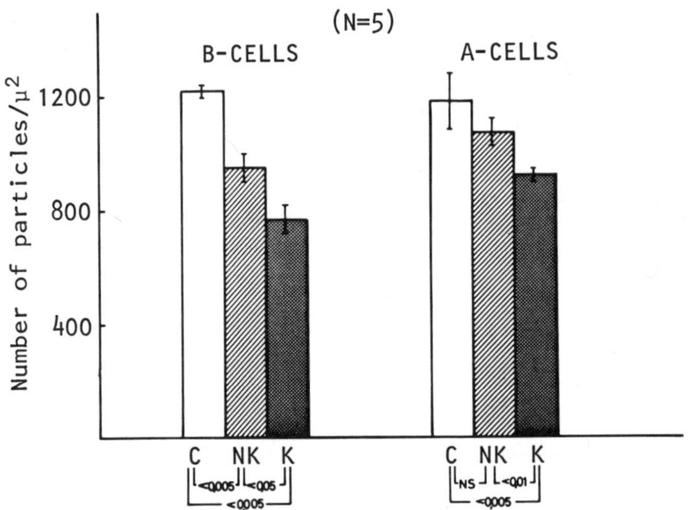

FIG. XXI. Number ($\pm$ SEM) of membrane-associated particles/μ^2 of plasma membrane (A-face) in B- and A-cells of control (C), diabetic (NK) and ketotic (K) Chinese hamsters. Also indicated is the statistical significance of the observed differences (NS = not significant).

particles in the plasma membrane was detectable and paralleled the
severity of the diabetic state: the difference between extreme values
corresponded to a 35% drop below control level. A similar, though
less marked trend was seen in the A cells. Associated with these
changes, we also noticed a loss of the random distribution pattern
of membrane-associated particles: the particles in diabetic animals
tended to be grouped in clusters (Figs. XXII, XXIII). Since experimental data are not yet available concerning the factors which control the distribution and size of membrane particles in general, one
cannot explain the significance of the changes described in islet
cells. Fusion of mobile particles within the fluid membrane matrix,
removal or decreased synthesis of membrane particles, preferential
insertion of membrane components lacking particles could account
for the changes noted respectively in the size, number and distribution of the particles. Although uninterpretable at the moment,
our observations clearly show that subtle changes in the ultrastructural organization of islet cells membrane are taking place in
the natural course of spontaneous diabetes mellitus in Chinese hamsters, and that these changes are not identical in A and B cells.
Beside the gross composition of the membrane, as it is reflected
morphologically in freeze-fracture, other factors could play a role
in the regulation of the activity of A and B cells. Such factors
are the intercellular junctions which
Alpha-beta cell   allow cells not only to communicate
coupling   one with another but also to modify the
                       permeability of the intercellular space
(for review, see ref. 85). Intercellular communication is one of
the basic prerequisites for the normal functioning of multicellu-
lar organisms and it is thought that communication (or coupling)
arises through the exchange of substances from one cell to another
(for review, see ref. 8). Circumstantial evidence accumulated over
the last few years points to a specific type of intercellular junction, the gap junction (116), as responsible for cell-to-cell coupling which can involve ions (ionic coupling) or small molecules
(metabolic coupling) (48, 63, 107 for review see ref. 85). Another specific junction, the tight junction (39) would be responsible for restricting the permeability of the intercellular space
(for review, see ref. 85). In gap junctions, the intercellular
space is narrowed to a 20-30 angstrom slit which has been shown to
be bridged by hydrophilic channels ensuring the movement of substances from one cell to another without loss in the intercellular
space. In tight junctions the intercellular space is completely
obliterated by the fusion of the outer leaflets of the two adjacent
cell membranes. In islet cells, the only intercellular junction
which was recognized for a long time was the desmosome (Fig. XXIVA)
(implicated in cell-to-cell adhesion) and it is only recently that
we succeeded in identifying both gap and tight junctions between
these cells (102, 103) (for review see ref. 94). As intramembranous specializations, these latter are best seen in freeze-fracture

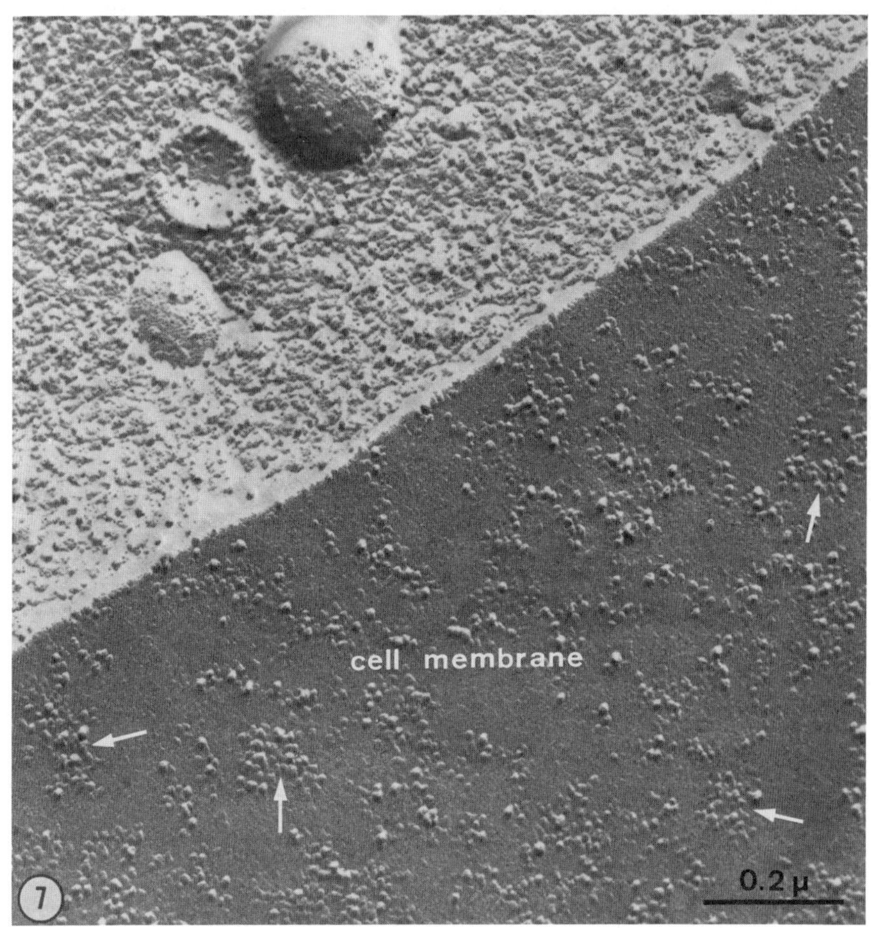

FIG. XXII. B-cell of diabetic Chinese hamster.
Most of the particles in the membrane face are
grouped in clusters (arrows). Compare with
Fig. XVIII.

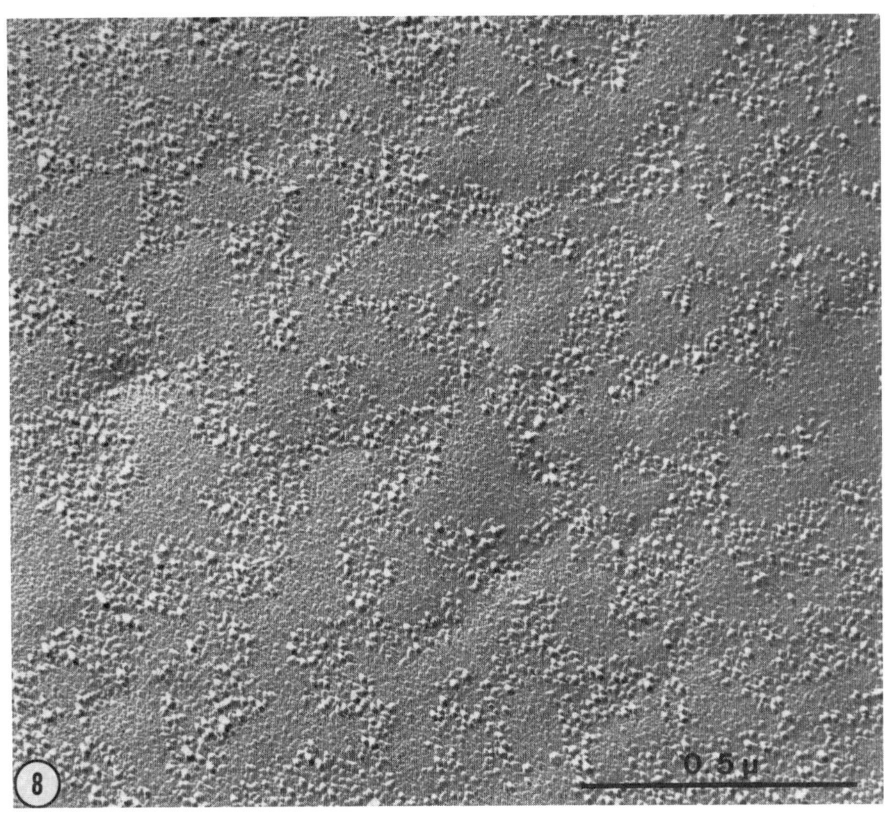

FIG. XXIII. B-cell of diabetic (ketotic) Chinese
hamster. The clusters of particles in the membrane
face are separated by relatively smooth areas.

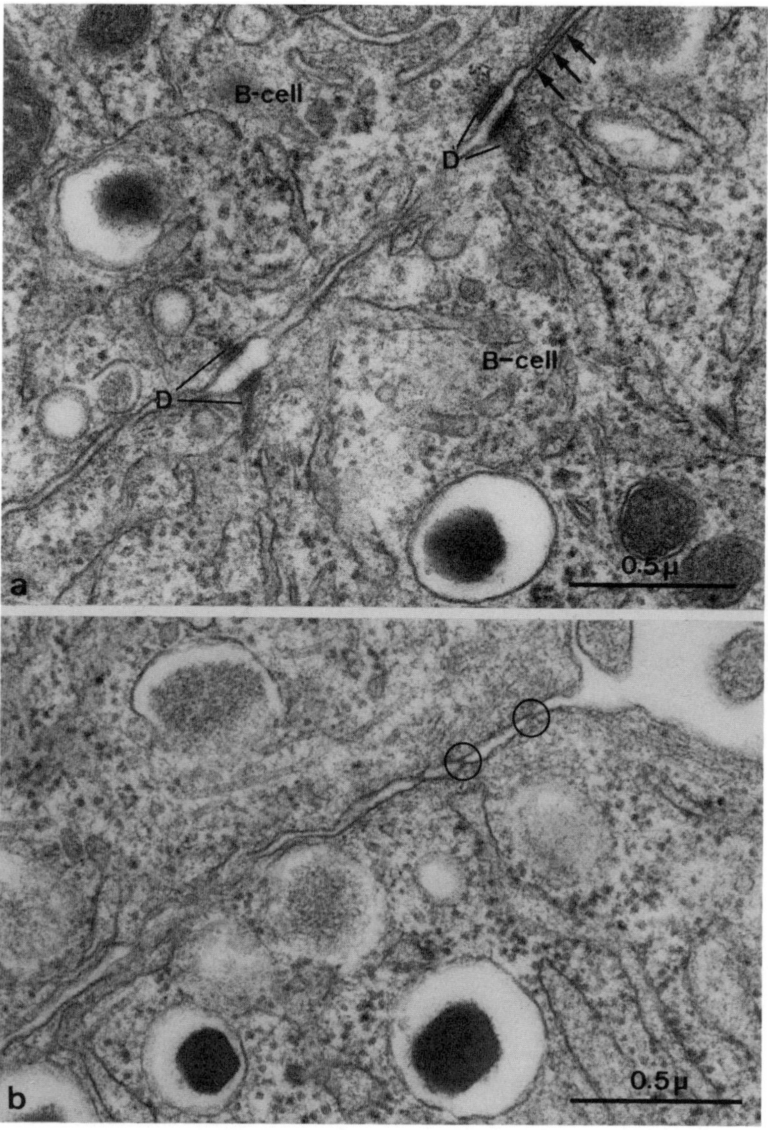

FIG. XXIV. B-cells of the rat. Thin section.
(a) The intercellular space is enlarged at the sites
of desmosomes (D) which are characterized additionally
by a densification of the cytoplasm beneath the plasma
membranes. Desmosomes have an adhesive function. The
arrows point to another type of cell contact in which
the intercellular space appears considerably narrowed
(presumably a nexus or gap junction).
(b) The encircled areas indicate the regions where the
intercellular space seems focally obliterated (presumably by a tight junction.

replicas (70): tight junctions are seen as ridges or fibrils in
the membrane face, whereas gap junctions consist of aggregates of
closely packed membrane particles. As shown in Fig. XXV, well-
defined fibrils characterizing tight junctions are constantly found
in B-cells membranes. The extent and complexity of such elements
is variable and it can be modified experimentally, for example by
exposure of isolated islets in vitro to proteolytic enzymes (95-99
for review see ref 94). This treatment increases dramatically
the length of tight junctional elements as seen in freeze-fracture
replicas (Figs. XXVI, XXVII).

We have recently been able to examine in freeze-fracture,
islets from human pancreas. As shown
Human Data   in Fig. XXVIII, the preparations show
                               a profusion of tight junctional elements.
We explain this increase by the fact that there is a relatively long
interval (1-3 hours) of time elapsed between the mincing of the
pancreatic tissue and the completion of islet isolation, during
which islets are certainly exposed to proteases from damaged acinar
cells. We have mentioned above the effect of proteolytic enzymes
on the development of tight junctions. Moreover, when islets of
rat are isolated in the same conditions as human islets, a comparable increase in tight junctions can be produced (98). The fact
that such junctions can be modified experimentally clearly indicates
that they are highly labile differentiations, and probably reflects
their ability to constantly modulate intercellular relationships.

Fig. XXIX shows the membrane differentiation characteristic
of the gap junction, as it appears on islet cell membrane. As previously demonstrated in other tissues, gap junctions appear as aggregates of regularly packed particles, which have the additional characteristic of being very regular in both shape and size within the
aggregates. Another aspect of islet junctions elucidated by freeze-
fracture is the frequent association of gap junctions with elements
of tight junctions (Figs. XXX-XXXII). In general, one can say that
it is the small size of both tight and gap junctions which renders
it difficult to show them in thin section (Fig. XXIVB). However, it
is the latter technique, on material treated with lanthanum so as to
blacken the extracellular space, which allowed us to show that such
junctions occurred not only between B-cells but also between A and
B cells (Fig. XXXIII). Since gap junctions are considered to provide
diffusion channels for ions and molecules up to 500 MW (8) from
one cell to another and that gap junctions seem to be widespread
between islet cells, one can consider an islet as a large functional
syncytium working as a single multihormonal unit. These findings
thus provide a morphological basis for the concept that A and B cells
could act synergistically, releasing precisely titrated quantities
of secretory products that are in physiologic opposition to each other
and yet maintain extracellular glucose concentration within a tightly

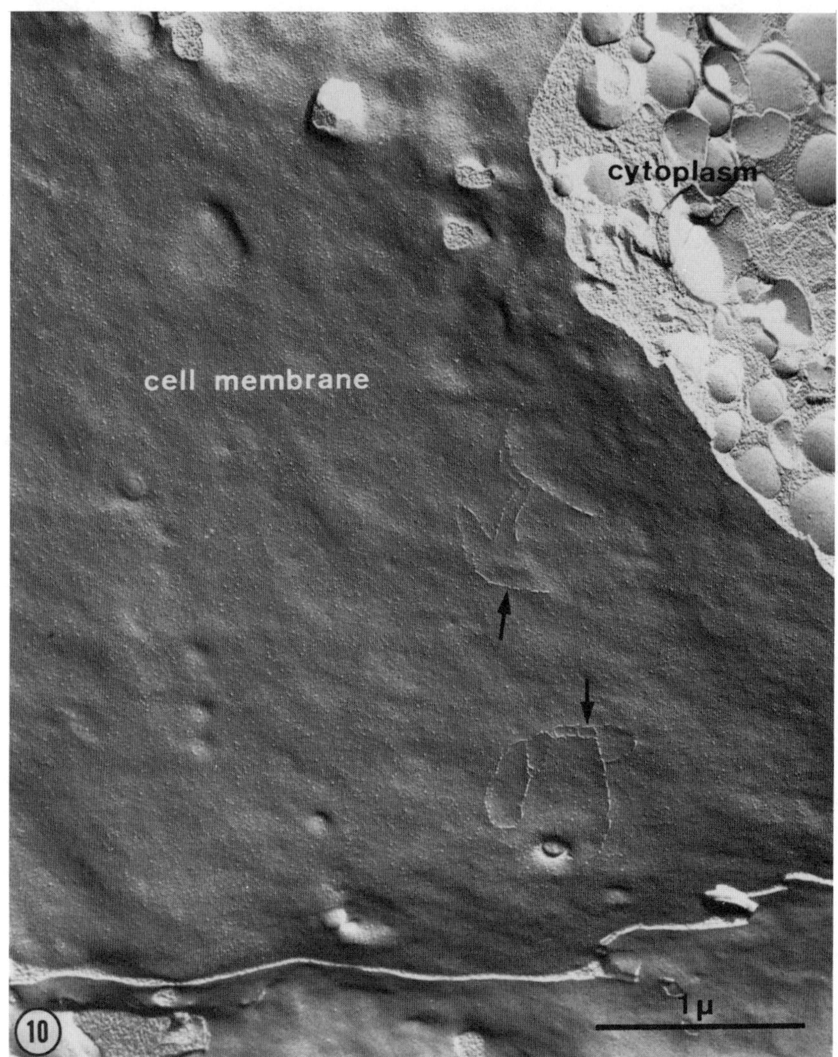

FIG. XXV. Islet cells of the rat. Freeze-fracture.
Both cell membrane and cytoplasm have been exposed.
In the cell membrane, one distinguishes linear ridges
or fibrils which represent tight junctions (arrows).

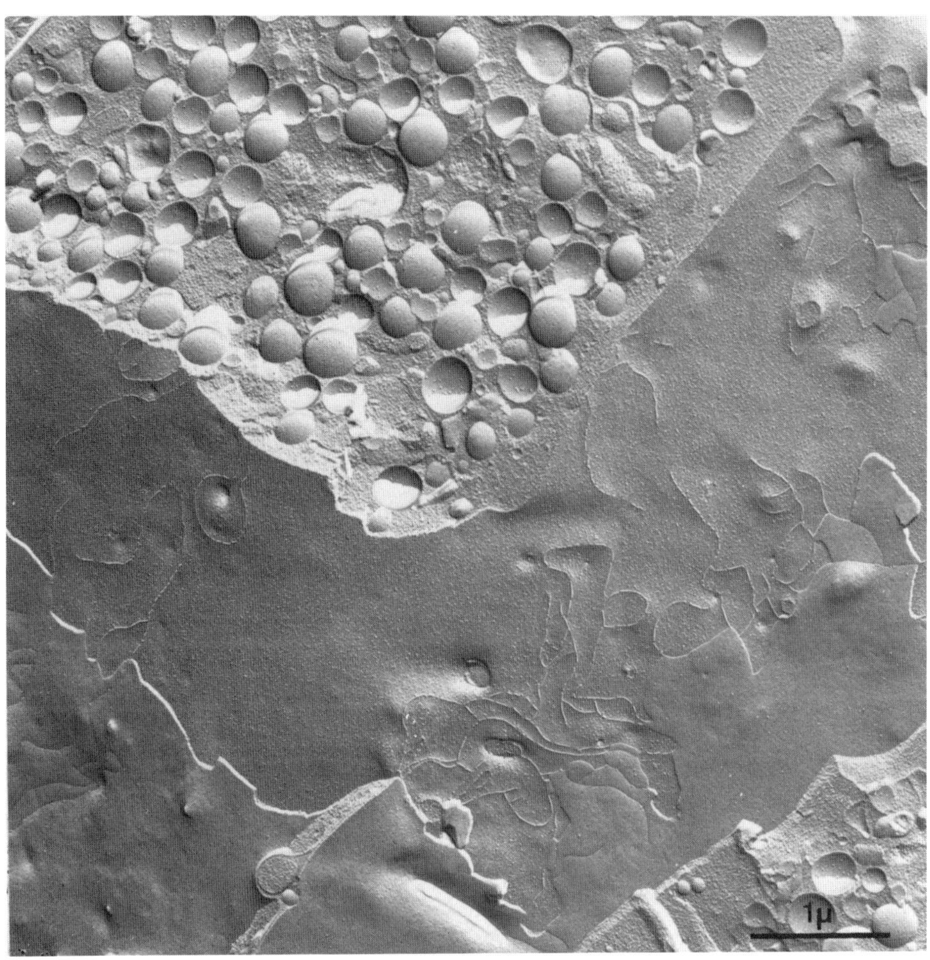

FIG. XXVI. Rat islet cells. Freeze-fracture. In
this case the islet was treated with pronase (4 µg/ml)
for 90 minutes before freeze-fracturing. Numerous
tight junctional elements are present in the cell
membrane.

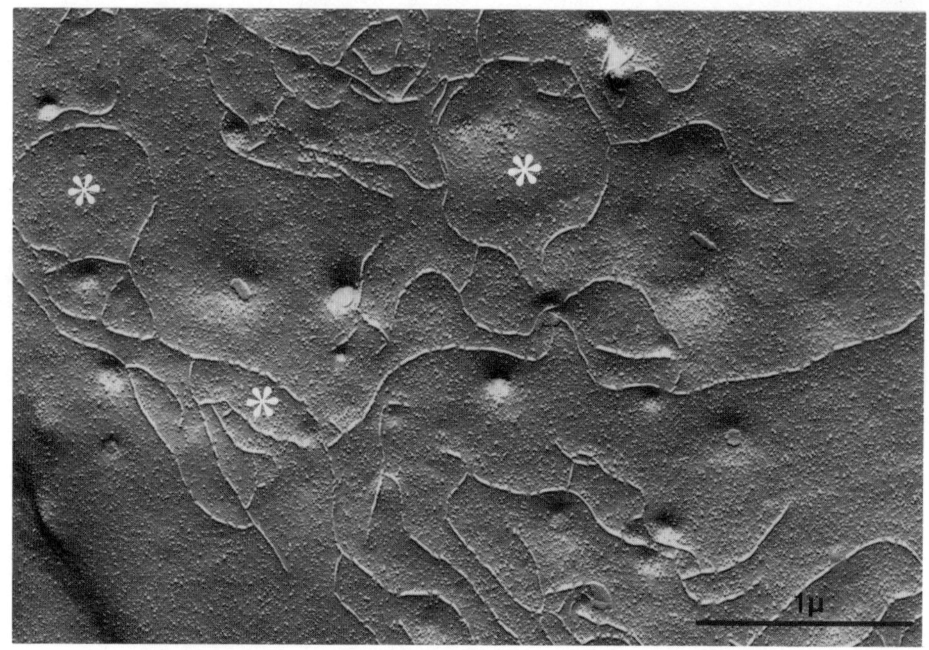

FIG. XXVII. Rat islet cells. Freeze-fracture.
Treatment of the islet with pancreatic proteases
(Sigma type I) (10 μg/ml) for 90 minutes induced
the formation of an extensive and ramified net-
work of tight junctional fibrils in the membrane
face.

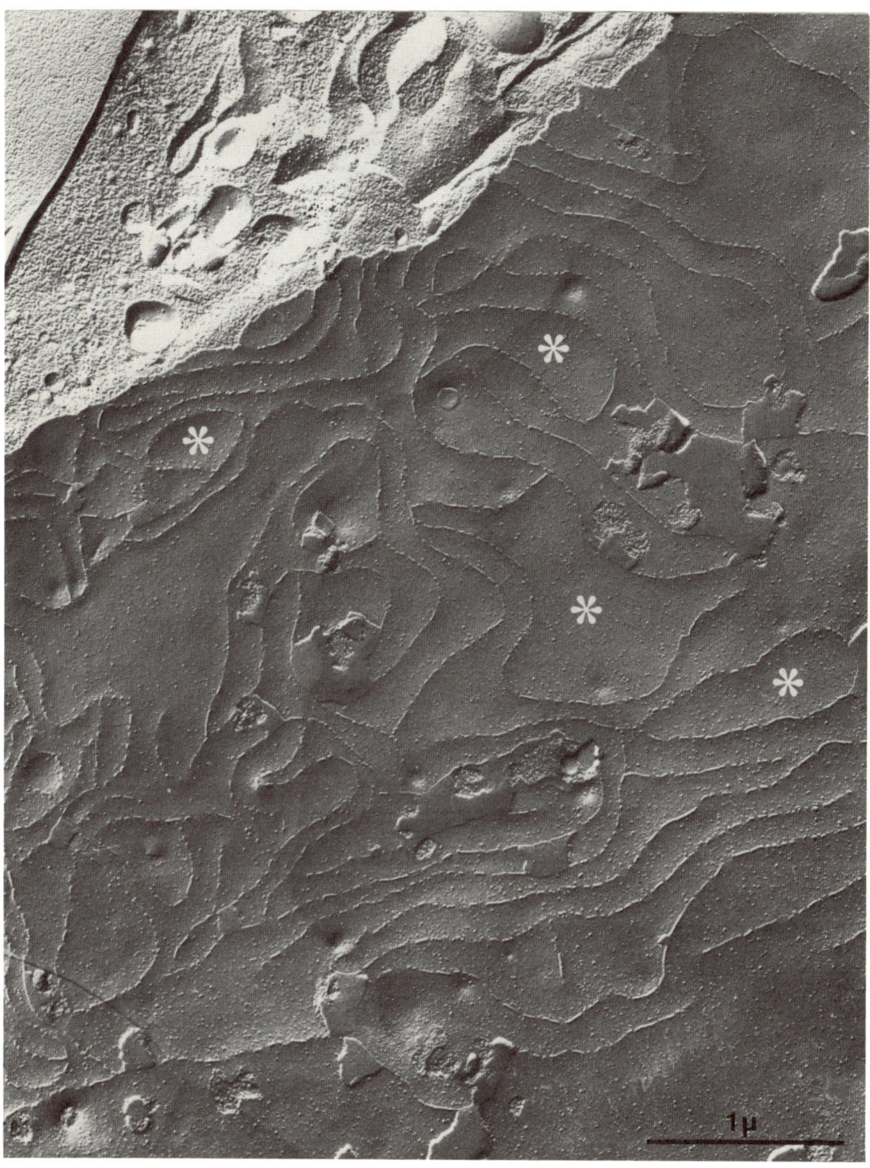

FIG. XXVIII. Human islet cells. Freeze-fracture.
The tight junctional elements (fibrils) involve a
large area of the cell membrane and delineates a
series of closed domains (asterisks) within the
junctional region. Such a development of the
tight junctions could have been caused by pancreatic
proteases leaking from damaged exocrine cells during
the time elapsed (3 h) between the mincing of the
pancreas and the completion of islets isolation.

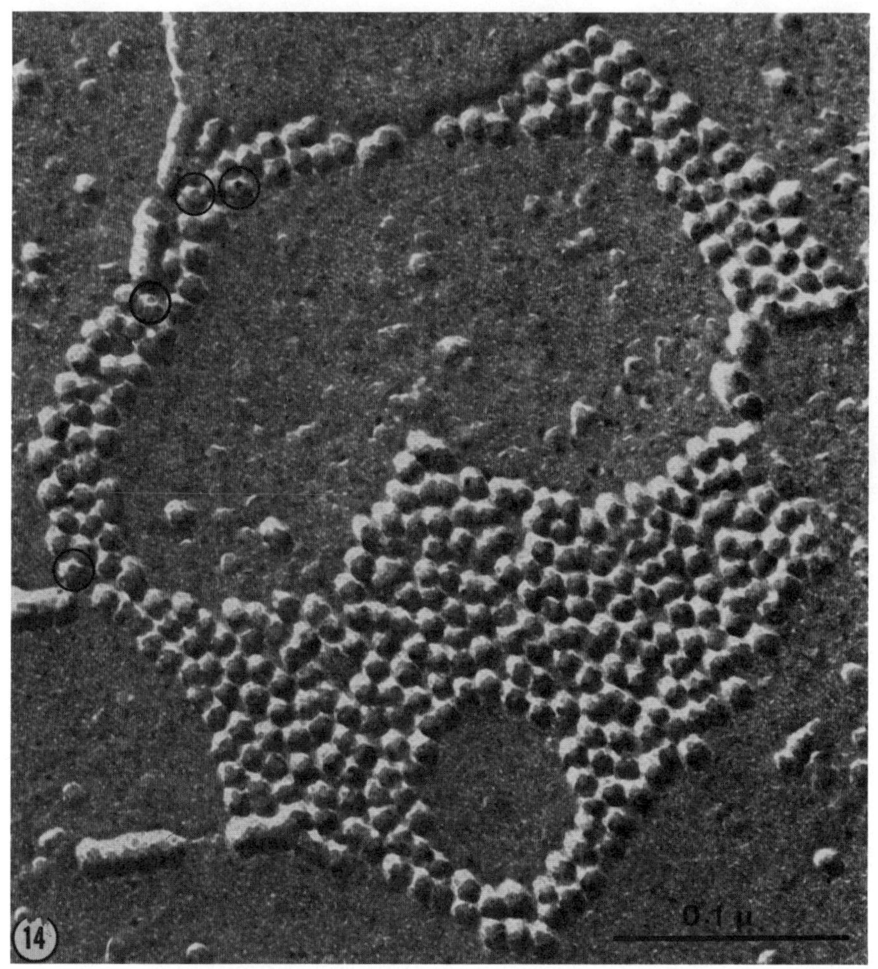

FIG. XXIX. Rat islet cell. Freeze-fracture.
This highly organized aggregate of particles
in the membrane face corresponds to a nexus
(gap junction). A close scrutiny of the aggregate
reveals that the particles have a polygonal shape
and that a pit (channel?) is visible on some of
them (circles).

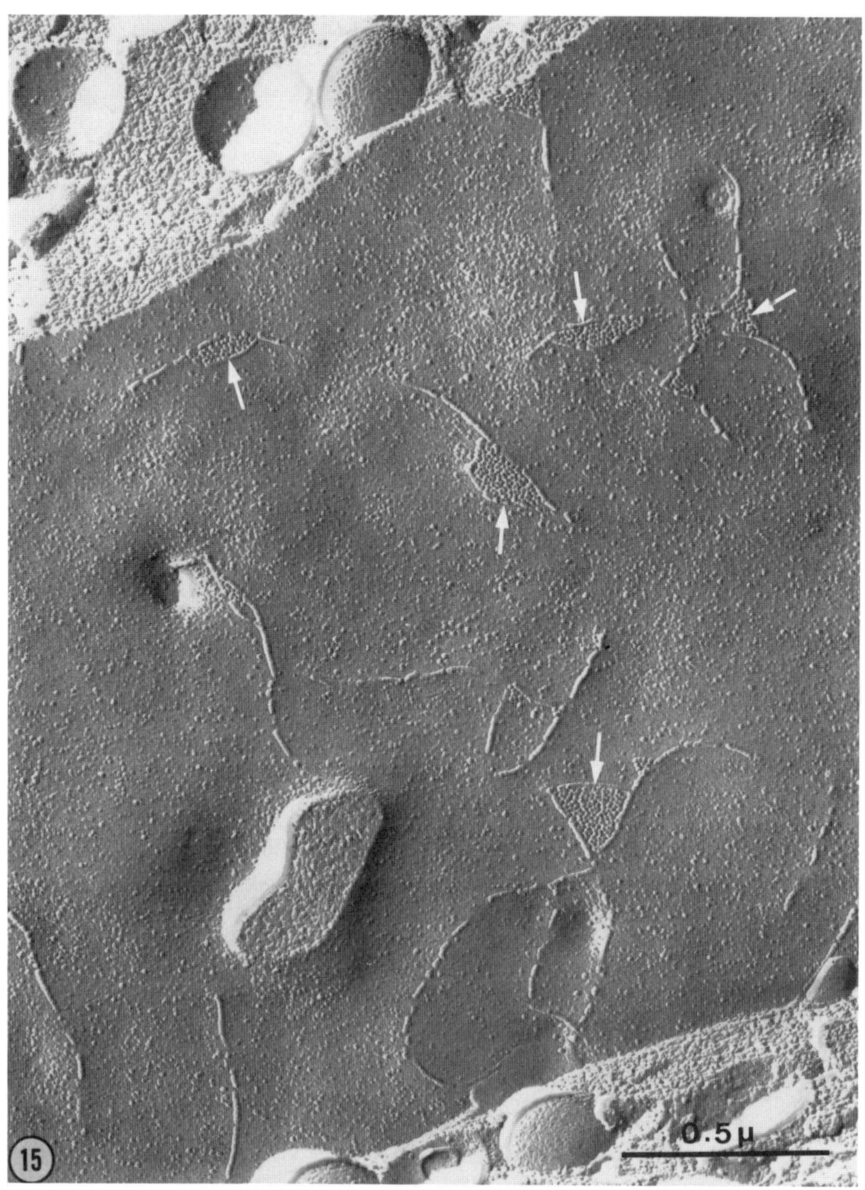

FIG. XXX. Rat islet cell. Freeze-fracture.
The membrane face contains several aggregates
of particles characteristic of gap junctions
associated with tight junctions fibrils (arrows).

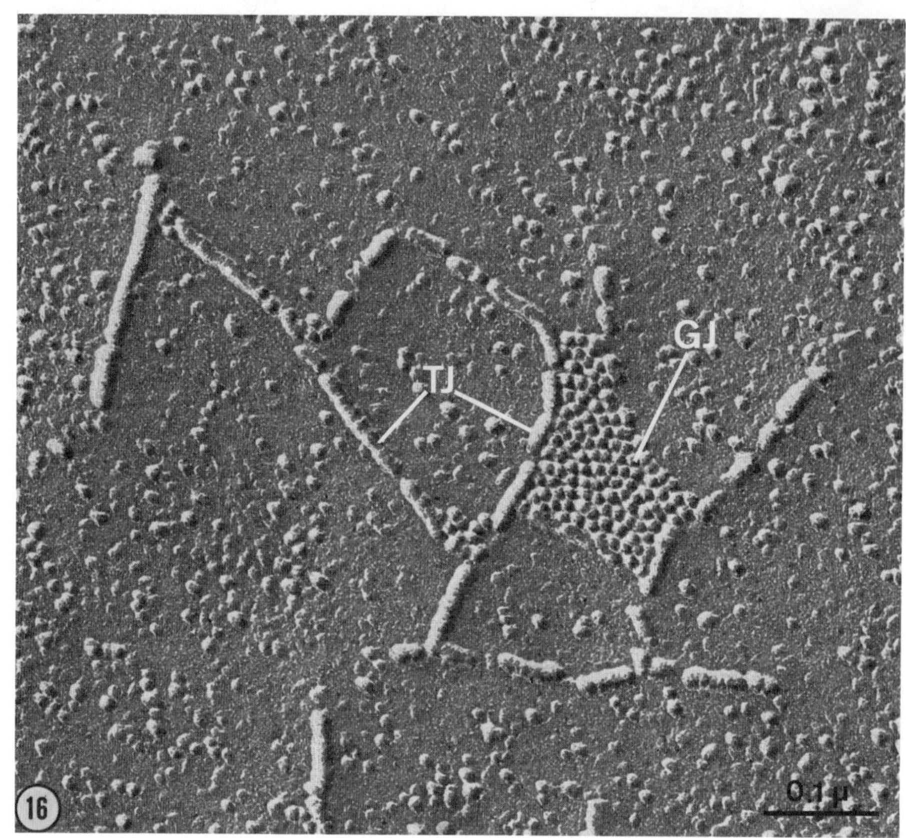

FIG. XXXI. Rat islet cell. Freeze-fracture.
The close association between gap junctions (GJ)
and tight junctions (TJ) is visible. The regularity in size of the closely packed particles forming
the gap contrasts with the various diameters of
the particles outside the junctional area.

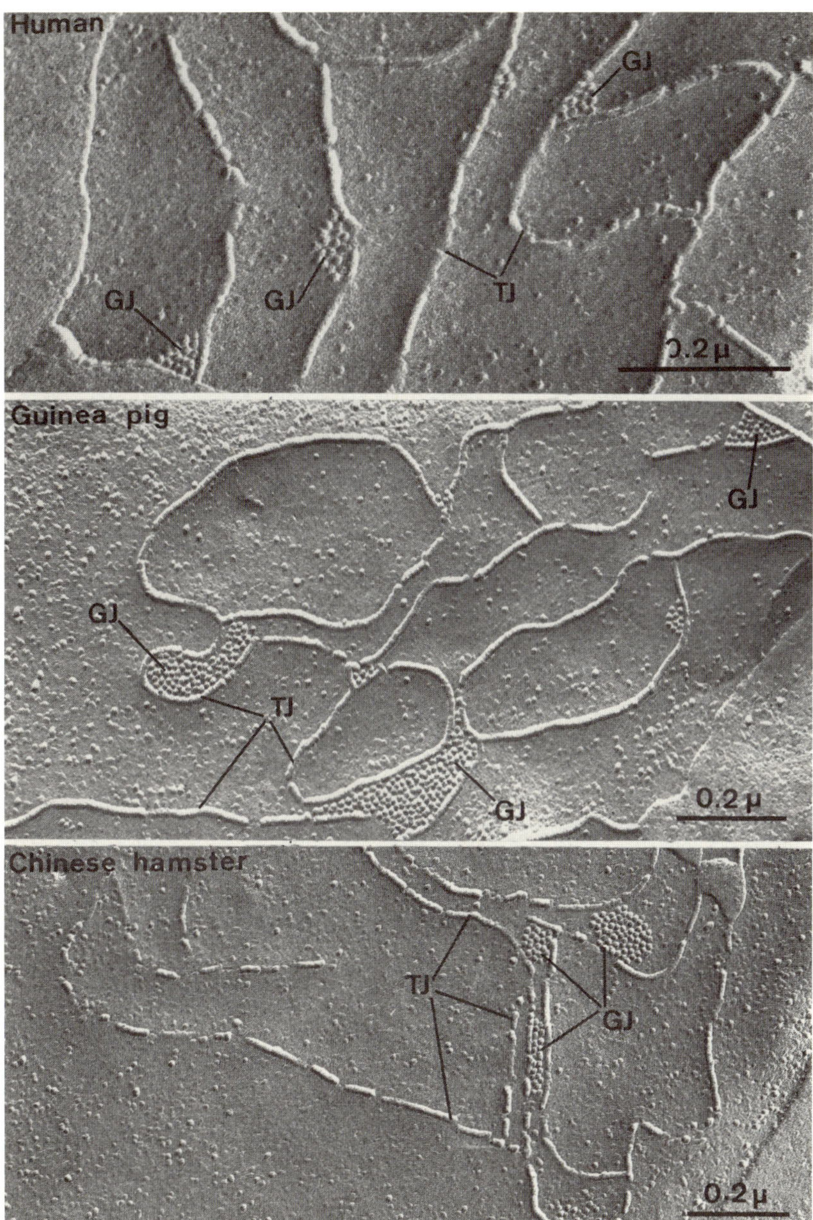

FIG. XXXII. Freeze-fracture replicas comparing the morphological appearance of tight (TJ) and gap junctions (GJ) in different mammalian species. In all three examples shown here, the association of tight junctional fibrils with gap junctional aggregates of particles is present.

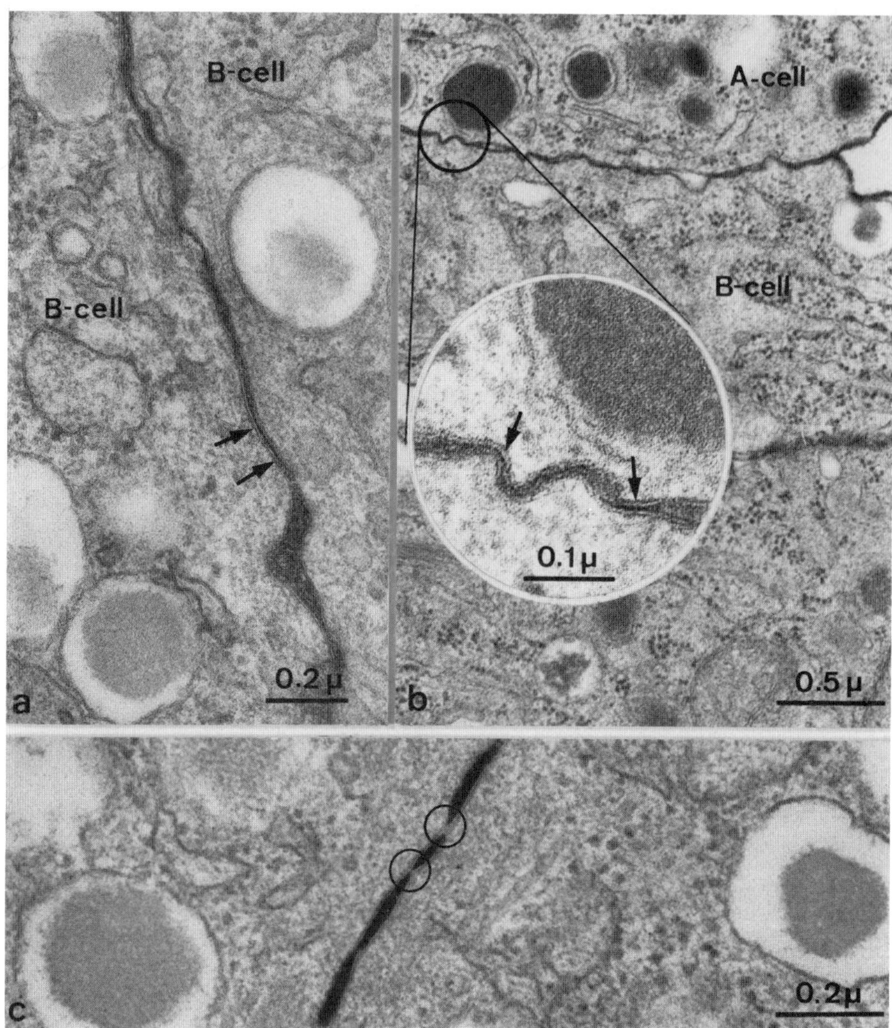

FIG. XXXIII. Rat islet cells. Thin section. The
preparation was treated with lanthanum hydroxyde which
delineates the intercellular space in black. At the
levels indicated by the arrows, one can observe focal
narrowings of the intercellular space (a and b). In
these regions, which probably represent gap junctions,
the intercellular space seems to maintain an uniform
width (~40 angstrom). In c, the lanthanum fills the
intercullular space up to the region (see encircled areas)
in which converging membranes fuse to form focal tight
junctions. The tracer is excluded from such junctions.

constricted range during major changes in glucose turnover.

In conclusion, I hope that my presentation has convinced you that the shift in morphological technique from thin-sectioning to freeze-fracturing has opened a new field in the study of cellular membranes and thereby places the morphologist in a position to address himself to problems concerning function which were out of his reach not so long ago.

DR. SPRITZ: I would like to ask you a question about the first part of your presentation, about those nuclear pores and the differences that are shown in the diabetic animal. These, I take it, were the beta cells and the alpha cells also, in these hamsters that developed diabetes. Do you have any information about whether this is specific for the islet cells or whether this is an effect of the diabetes, which would be found in other cells?

DR. ORCI: So far, we have performed this study only on isolated islets.

DR. SPRITZ: Do you have enough animals to show the results following treatment with insulin? That is, to get a ketoacidotic animal that is treated and then see what were the possible changes following treatment?

DR. ORCI: All animals studied were untreated, but we hope to perform the same study in treated animals later. Unfortunately, these animals do not seem to appreciate the comfort of Kalamazoo-Geneva flights and they need continuous nursing.

DR. WILLIAMS: I suppose you have not yet looked at any cells from a streptozotocinized as well as alloxanized animals?

DR. ORCI: We have performed preliminary studies on the effect of streptozotocin and alloxan on the islet cells of spiny mice (96). A dramatic drop in the number of intramembranous particles was noticed 10 minutes after the administration of alloxan and 60 minutes after streptozotocin injection. It should be stressed that these changes occurred at times known to be characterized by a marked impairment of secretory capacity of B cells.

DR. CAHILL: After the administration of the alloxan, did you see any further changes in the cell structure?

DR. ORCI: There seemed also to be a change in the <u>distribution</u> of the particles as a result of both alloxan and streptozotocin administration. The decreased density of particles is accompanied by a loss of their random distribution, large areas of plasma membrane being virtually devoid of particles, or presenting particles grouped in clusters of various sizes.

DR. WILLIAMS: It might be interesting to observe the effect of adding insulin antibody to your culture after you have exposed the culture to this for an hour or two and then to see what it does to the surface areas.

DR. ORCI: Thank you for your suggestion.

DR. WILLIAMS: How about the interconnecting mechanism?

DR. ORCI: The demonstration that gap junctions ensure a communication between adjacent cells has been done in cultured cells, using a combination of ultrastructural, electrophysiological and dye-injection techniques (63). Whenever adjacent cells were metabolically coupled, electrically coupled or that fluorescein injected into one cell passed on to the other, it was possible to demonstrate a gap junction between them. This type of experiment has yet to be done on islet cells.

Alpha-beta cell relationship in cell cultures

DR. SPRITZ: How specific are these ridges that you see between beta cells and between beta and alpha cells which you referred to? Do most adjacent cells do this? Is this found in other tissues? Or does this have a special implication to the pancreatic cells? I want to get a feeling of how common this phenomenon is throughout the cells of the entire organism.

DR. ORCI: Tight junctions are quite frequent in many kinds of cells, and are characteristically developed in anatomical areas where physical compartmentalization of the intercellular space is important.

DR. WOLF: Dr. Orci, you said that the extent of tight junctions varies from time to time.

DR. ORCI: Yes, it is true, and this means to us that these structures are not stable. If they had a definite structure, we would always see them in one form. In fact, they are able to change under certain circumstances. If you expose islets to pancreatic proteases, within one hour a very extensive development of tight junctions occurs. Incidentally, this raises again the old question: why are islets scattered throughout exocrine pancreas?

Rearrangement of junctional connections

DR. CAHILL: It appears to be a question of a random happening. One might say that they just happened there.

DR. ORCI: Why is it then, that if the parathyroid gland, the
pituitary or the adrenal medulla are exposed to pancreatic enzymes,
one does not observe a development of tight junctional elements?
Is the capability to develop tight junctions an inherent characteristic of islet cells as such, or do they acquire the susceptibility
to develop these junctions by their proximity to exocrine tissue?

DR. UNGER: Dr. Orci, have you looked at cells for some differences that may relate from the viewpoint of a specific location
in the exocrine tissue, or can't you isolate the cells with that
degree of specificity?

DR. ORCI: In many mammalian species, the islets of Langerhans
are surrounded by a shell of distinctive acini. These acini are
composed of large cells packed with zymogen granules. In the spiny
mice (Acomys cahirinus) the periinsular exocrine shell remains
attached to the islets during the procedure of islet isolation with
collagenase. In collaboration with F. Malaisse-Lagae and W. J.
Malaisse, we have used this animal model to investigate the possible
heterogeneity between periinsular and non-periinsular (or teleinsular) exocrine pancreas. This was tested by measuring hydrolase
concentrations in homogenates of small fragments of teleinsular
tissue and of islets with attached periinsular tissue. In order
to correct for the variable amount of exocrine tissue present in
each sample, we have expressed the concentrations of amylase, lipase
and chemotrypsinogen relative to each other. It was thus found that
the pattern of hydrolase content was different in the two exocrine
tissue compartments, the concentration of amylase relative to that
of lipase, for example, being invariably higher in the teleinsular
than in the periinsular acini. The possibility that such a functional compartmentation of the exocrine pancreas also exists in other
mammals is now under investigation in our laboratory.

DR. CAHILL: But the random distribution is limited only to the
mammals; when you get to the birds, one sees separate types of islet
cells.

DR. ORCI: I do not think that animals exist which have completely separate locations for A and B cells: in birds, dark and
light islets only show a predominance of A cells and B cells, respectively.

DR. SPRITZ: Have you studied any fetal pancreas? My question
                          is: can there be a stage where there
Fetal development   is only endocrine tissue and no exocrine
of pancreatic cells   tissue?

DR. ORCI: During fetal development, as soon as pancreatic endocrine tissue is recognizable as such, exocrine cells are also present.

DR. LEVINE: Roger Unger referred in the past to "the embryo-
logical time appearance of alpha versus beta secretory material".
As I used to hear it there seemed to be a tremendous difference
in time but now there seems to be a tendency to diminish this
difference. I would like to know what is the present situation?

DR. UNGER: Well, that is true. Glucagon appears very early,
but what is interesting is that glucagon receptors in the liver
do not appear that early. This is work that is going on right now
in our laboratory.

DR. LEVINE: But isn't it true that insulin appears in the
blood earlier?

DR. CAHILL: But glucagon appears in 8 to 10 weeks in man.

DR. WOLF: The phylogenetic approach including the study of
primitive marine vertebrates may prove illuminating. The cyclo-
stomes, hagfish and lamprey, appear to possess insulin secreting
beta cells but no alpha cells and no glucagon. Alpha cells and
glucagon first make their appearance among teleosts. It may therefore be possible to establish as a baseline the insulin regulatory
mechanisms that obtain prior to the appearance of glucagon in the
course of biological evolution.

DR. ORCI: Dr. Like and myself have reported that, in human
embryos, only A cells are identified at 9 weeks of gestation. At
10.5 weeks, D and B cells are also present (77).

DR. WOLF: You did not say anything about the other cells in
the islets. Do you have some data on that?

DR. ORCI: As to the other cells, I cannot say anything at
present. I have data only on the A cells and the B cells. However,
it would be possible to collect data on D cell membrane too, since,
in the Chinese hamster, the D cells can be identified because of the
polymorphism of their secretory granules. So far the number of
D cells encountered in freeze-fracture preparations was too small
to allow any quantification of morphological parameters as we did
for A and B cells.

DR. WILLIAMS: Vascular abnormalities cause far more difficulty
in diabetes than does ketoacidosis. They consist of microangiopathies and precocious atherosclerosis. The former accounts for
most of the deaths in juvenile-onset diabetics, and the latter for
most of those in adult-onset diabetics. Microangiopathy is present
in the majority of diabetics previous to the development of demonstrable glucose intolerance (126), and progresses in spite of
careful therapy. Capillaries of skeletal muscles, skin, kidney,
retina and other organs are involved (140-143). Characteristically the basal lamina is not diffusely thickened but consists of
excessive investment of multiple apposing layers (see Fig. XXXIV).
Similar reduplication of basal lamina can be produced in normoglycemic animals by killing cells and letting the injury heal.
Newly formed cells repopulate the pre-existing basal lamina scaf-
folds and deposit a new layer of basal lamina in apposition to the
old one. It appears that each layer of basal lamina represents
the residual evidence of one cell generation and that the excessive
accumulation of basal lamina in diabetes suggests that cells are
dying and replenished at an accelerated rate. These microvascular
changes are found to occur in markedly different degrees in various
portions of the body. There are three anatomical sites in which
excessive basal lamina accumulation are especially pertinent in
diabetes: (a) retinal capillaries with microaneurysms developing
at sites in which mural cells (pericytes) have degenerated and
presumably caused weakness in the vessel wall; (b) a diffuse type
of accumulation of basal lamina, causing diffuse capillary glomerulosclerosis and accumulations in the mesangium, and diffuse and
nodular intercapillary glomerulosclerosis; and (c) a reduplication
of the basal lamina in the Schwann cells.

In studies of skin fibroblast cultures, Vracko and Benditt
found that the rate of cell death and cell replenishment was
accelerated in diabetics, but there was a decrease in the total
number of doublings, in comparison with cells from nondiabetics
(142). These investigators suggested that there is a decreased
replicative lifespan of diabetic fibroblasts in vitro, and that
this is an expression of increased susceptibility of these cells
to injury and dying. They regarded this as a genetically transmitted defect in all cells in the body. Although accumulation of
basal lamina is not specific for diabetes but occurs with aging
and other processes, the authors did not regard the changes in
diabetes as a manifestation of aging.

Since most diabetic patients eventually show characteristic
microangiopathy and changes in the pancreatic islets, the question
is often posed as to whether: (a) microvascular changes lead to

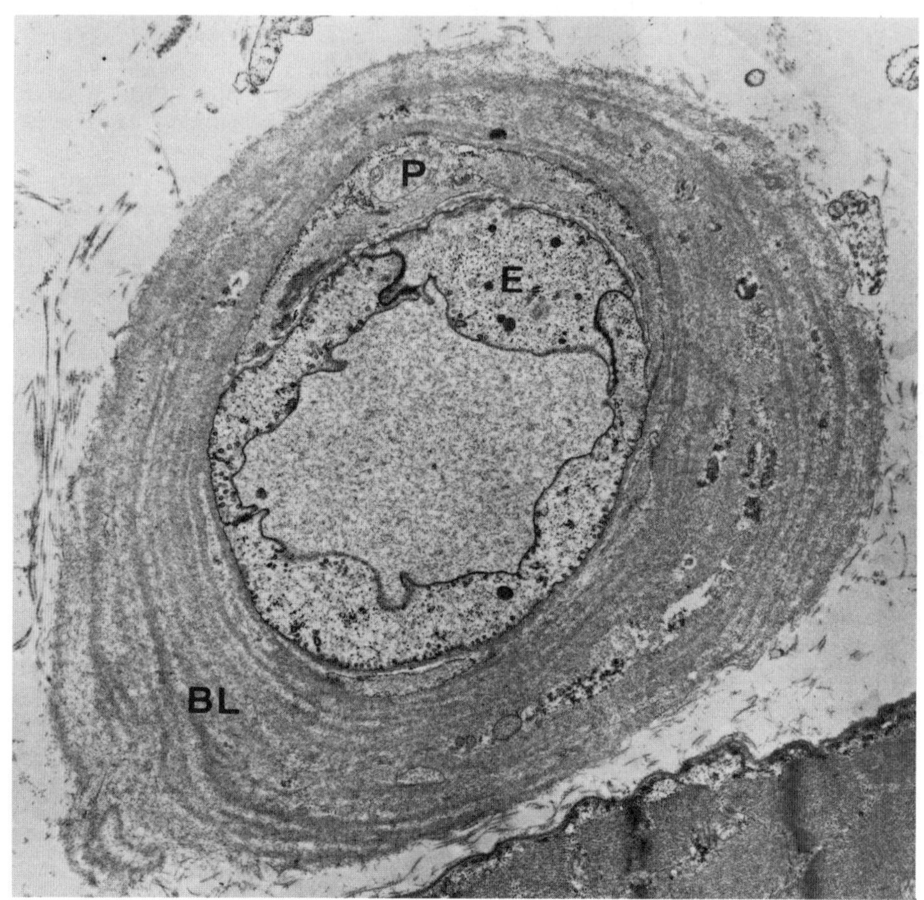

FIG. XXXIV. Cross-section of capillary from plantar
muscle from a patient, aged 70, who had been known to
have diabetes for 20 years (X 7,350). The lumen, endothelial cell (E) and pericyte (P) are surrounded by
multiple layers of basal lamina (BL), between which
cellular debris is present. The pericyte is separated
from the endothelial cell by a single, normally thick
layer of basal lamina. The many basal lamina appear
like growth rings of a tree. (After Vracko & Benditt).

the alterations in the islet cell activities; (b) the alterations
in islets lead to the microvascular changes; or (c) some factor
causes both the microvascular and islet cell changes (143). The
following are among the reasons why some investigators conclude
that alterations in islet cell activities do not cause microvascular
changes: (a) Siperstein reported that 74% of prediabetics that he
examined had thickening of the basement membrane (126) (prediabetics
do not have elevated plasma glucose); (b) the amount of microvascular alteration is not proportionate to the duration or amount of
hyperglycemia; (c) islet destruction (alloxan, pancreatitis) or
removal (surgical) has been reported not to produce the complete
diabetic syndrome. However, it should be emphasized that most
diabetes is apparently due to a genetic disorder, and biochemical
abnormalities exist since before birth. Abnormalities in the net
function of insulin could lead to numerous alterations in different
parts of the body. As discussed earlier, the amount of plasma
insulin activity can influence the number of insulin receptors on
certain body cells. Moreover, the age at which abnormalities are
produced can have an enormous influence on the net biochemical and
histological changes that develop. Many of the experimental models
that have had removal or destruction of the islets were at ages
long past birth. We know that a given amount of hormonal change
can have enormous influence in utero or soon after birth, but will
have relatively minor effects at a much later stage in life.

I do not find good evidence that the vascular changes cause
the islet damage. However, one can
visualize a type of genetic abnormality
The mechanism of basement
membrane thickening - the
pericyte
that could cause alterations in fibroblasts and other cells of the body as
well as in the islet cells.

The factor causing alterations in the germ plasm could be any
one of several types -- a viral infection or various chemicals.
Moreover, autoimmune disease could account for both the vascular
changes and the islet changes and also be on the basis of genetic
changes.

DR. KNOWLES: Dr. Williams has mentioned the pericyte and discussed its possible involvement in the pathological process of
microvascular disease. Since about 1961, at the Cherry Hill Conference on microangiopathy, experts on electronmicroscopy have had
very different opinions as to what was a pericyte (76). Last
year, I had the opportunity to listen to the same people, and there
still seemed to be difficulty in deciding what was a pericyte.

DR. ORCI: I would like to stress that there is a very close
resemblance between the mesangial cell of the kidney glomerulus
and the pericytes (or Rouget cells) of capillaries elsewhere in

the body. One should remember that a pericyte is always inserted
almost totally within the split capillary basement membrane, and
in that manner it can establish a close relationship with the
endothelium through fine processes.

DR. KNOWLES: Well, Lelio, can you differentiate very easily
between the two?

DR. ORCI: Quite easily! A pericyte can be identified from
other cells because of its spatial relationships and its important
filamentous web.

DR. KNOWLES: I listened to a discussion a year ago where
there were doubts as to whether or not this was a pericyte or the
residue of a pericyte or an endothelial cell.

DR. WOLF: Lelio, what is the origin of pericytes? Do they
come from the endothelial cells?

DR. ORCI: I am unable to answer this question.

DR. CAHILL: Spiro found an increase in one of the enzymes
involved in the synthesis of the disaccharide unit which is found
in excess in human diabetic kidneys, when he studied kidney tissue
of rats with experimental diabetes (7). Unfortunately, he has
not looked at the glomerular tissue alone for this enzyme, which is
where the pathology occurs.

DR. KNOWLES: It should be possible to do because Beisswenger
has separated these out. (7)

DR. CAHILL: The capacity to isolate glomeruli for chemical
analysis is one thing. After sieving to obtain glomeruli, then
centrifugation, etc., enzyme activities might be expected to be
altered. Of course the real answer would be to culture glomeruli,
and Paul Beisswenger at Pennsylvania is trying to keep them going
in vitro for one to four days and then to look at them biochemically.
What Spiro found is that the activity of this enzyme tends to go
up in the insulin-deficient rat (131). Of course the real question is, "What controls the hydroxylation of the lysine itself?"
Because the excess disaccharide unit cannot be added until you
have an acceptor. It may not be just the carbohydrate related
enzyme because glucose-galactosyl-disaccharide cannot be added
unless there is acceptor hydroxylysine. A lot of work remains to
be done in this area to establish whether or not these extra
hydroxylysine-galactosyl-glucose moieties represent the key abnormality in basement membrane. Spiro speculates that the hygrosco-
pic nature of the disaccharide may result in altered permeability.

All cells, particularly those that get into trouble, such as the endothelial cell in chronic diabetes "see" the ambient concentraction of glucose. The glucose molecule itself (for which there is some precedent in the glycogen synthetic system) may alter reactions. Can hyperglycemia be the culprit?

We have heard a lot about Sorbitol and there is no question that when glucose is high, thanks to the very high Km of aldosereductase, sorbitol can accumulate in tissues.

The role of
Sorbitol

There is evidence that Sorbitol accumulates in the diabetic animal or man in spinal fluid, and also in peripheral nerve and in other tissues when blood glucose is high. There is no question that Sorbitol can cause the acute diabetes cataract in the experimental animal and very rarely in man (we see about one in every five years). I personally doubt whether an accumulation of Sorbitol has anything to do with other diabetic problems. We also feel it is unlikely that Sorbitol accumulations have anything to do with neuropathies seen in the mildest diabetic patients. An example is the 50 to 55 year old man with normal blood glucose or a minimal degree of hyperglycemia after his meals, who nevertheless has the flashing skin syndrome - a night-long burning skin sensation.

DR. SPRITZ: In terms of water transport, this amount of Sorbitol and fructose really constitutes very little water and its osmolar effect would be very low, about one milli-osmol.

DR. CAHILL: John Pappenheimer has just done some beautiful work on the rate of glucose transport into brain. Independent of insulin, the brain cell slowly equilibrates with the high glucose level outside of it. If you drop the glucose concentration water will move into the brain much faster than the glucose can equilibrate, so you therefore can have an edematous brain purely due to glucose. In fact you really have to invoke glucose in order to get the edema.

Let me move along now, back to the nerve. Most nonogenerians show classical mild sensory diabetic neuropathy, decreased sensations and decreased achilles reflexes. This suggests that the neuropathy could be simply an acceleration of the aging process of the nerves themselves or their associated cells. Spritz's findings suggest that aging neuropathy is indistinguishable from diabetic neuropathy and it is simply a matter of severity when it does occur. This fits in with what I think, namely that we are measuring a summation of phenomena. Thus, we have a diffuse mesenchymal disorder of some sort. I think that the work of Sam Goldstein, now updated, especially his studies on fibroblasts, contains the best data (50). But in the so-called "Hayflick" phenomenon in the

early 60s, Hayflick showed that if you take fibroblasts from young
people and put them in tissue culture, they will go just so many
generations (56). Then if you take fibroblasts from older people
there seems to be a built-in senescence, they do less well.

Goldstein, Soeldner and Littlefield took some of Soeldner's
patients, normals with strong diabetic
family histories, the same kind of
patient that Dr. Siperstein studied,
and grew their fibroblasts in tissue
culture. If their fibroblasts came from "prediabetic" twenty-
year-olds, they behaved like those taken from sixty-year olds (51).
This suggests that perhaps there is a primary cellular disorder in
the diabetic kindred which limits their life span, at least that
of their fibroblasts in tissue culture.

**Diabetes and
Aging**

DR. LEVINE: If you accept that, then you must say that a very
large number of mild diabetics of the older age group suffer from
a different disease.

DR. CAHILL: I think that is natural aging.

DR. LEVINE: Then it is not diabetes!

DR. CAHILL: Well, it is a matter of semantics.

DR. LEVINE: Agreed, it is a matter of semantics. Because if
a man lives to age 85 his fibroblast must have been doing all
right and he is just different from the other man.

DR. CAHILL: But at age 85 his fibroblast will have the same
built-in senescence as would be the case with the 25 year old
diabetic.

DR. LEVINE: That is right, but even if this man has hyperglycemia at 85 he is not the same kind of being that this younger
person is.

DR. CAHILL: That may be true. Observations indicate a large
incidence of atherosclerosis in the diabetic kindred which is completely divorced initially from the carbohydrate abnormality. The
implication is that diabetes may be a primary mesenchymal disorder
and that atherosclerosis may simply reflect a senescence of some
sort in the vascular intima and media. This all agrees with the
Vracko hypothesis that there is an earlier destruction of fibroblasts and a replacement by new ones and this results in an
increased turnover in these basement membranes (140). I honestly
believe that there is an inherent predisposition that has something
to do with a primary replicating disorder of the fibroblast and

perhaps other tissues of the body. The high correlation between
diabetes and other diseases related to deficient cellular replication, such as Fanconi's anemia, concurs with this hypothesis.
There are many other diseases, such as hemochromatosis, with a
disorder in iron transport. The incidence or prevalence of diabetes in relatives of patients with hemochromatosis greatly exceeds
that found in the normal population. So we are getting more and
more input into the hypothesis that there is some primary cellular
disorder underlying at least the atherosclerosis, perhaps also the
neuropathy. If a cell is more fragile, and if an abnormal metabolic milieu is added, such as hyperglycemia or uremia, one ampli-
fies the problems. This is the bugbear of the diabetic on a dialysis program whose atherosclerosis appears grossly accelerated.

DR. UNGER: The real question which has never been answered
in a satisfactory fashion, is whether
or not treating the glucose level or
other metabolic abnormalities of diabetes with insulin would spare the
diabetic patient the ravages of small
vessel disease. That is to say: which
comes first, the small vessel disease or the metabolic disorder?
It is the key question in diabetes and it is appalling that we
really do not have a good answer after all these years of study.
As far as the controversies that surround the questions of small
vessel disease, I feel that some of the arguments are spurious
and that they are non-arguments that can be disposed of because
they cloud the real arguments that cannot be disregarded. I am
referring to the debate as to how to quantitate the small vessel
lesions, that is the basement membrane lesions. And as Dr. Williams
pointed out, where you get the biopsy and what constitutes absolute
measurements are important elements. Siperstein's study in 1968
(126) showed that although the absolute measurements may vary
from one muscle to another, the relationships between diabetics
and non-diabetics hold with regard to the thickness of their res-
pective basement membranes. So I don't think that, in the type of
diabetes that we generally accept and call genetic diabetes, there
is much difference in what we consider as being a small vessel
lesion in muscle.

_Significance of
"control" of diabetes
to microvascular
lesions_

One point which has aroused a lot of unnecessary argument in
my opinion is whether one should mea-
sure the thickness of the basement
membrane as Marvin Siperstein does,
namely by putting a grid in a random
way around a capillary and then measur-
ing it at each point where the grid intersects the basement membrane.
Calibration is, of course, essential and this was taken into consideration in this work. Dr. Williamson argues that one should

_The assessment of
Capillary Basement
Membrane Thickening_

choose the narrowest part of the blood vessel arbitrarily and then
measure (146). Now as I recall, Williamson reports about 50%
and Siperstein reports 98% which would indicate the relative sen-
sitivities of the two methods. The argument that tangential cuts
vitiate this type of measurement does not hold. It is clear that
thickening of the basement membrane is characteristic of diabetes.
When one gets to the pre-diabetic, Dr. Williams has already pointed
out that one has to be extremely cautious. In the first place, the
differences between the pre-diabetic group and the normal group are
far less dramatic than the difference between the normal and the
diabetic group. Nevertheless, as Dr. Williams pointed out, Siperstein showed that approximately 78% of individuals with a single
normal glucose tolerance, and with two diabetic parents, have
measurements above 1,500 angstroms, which I believe is the cut-off
point.

DR. WOLF: Do you have any information with regard to how many
individuals in that group ultimately develop diabetes?

DR. UNGER: Yes. Siperstein has those data and he is report-
ing on them. However, the incidence during the first five years
after the initial visits was in the 30% range amongst those who
have been attending our laboratory (125). It was much lower
than in Dr. Soeldner's group.

The second question that has caused a great deal of dispute
is the matter of whether duration of diabetes and age increases the
size of the thickening of the basement membrane and here again, I
don't see that this is a very important argument for this reason.
We know that with time microangiopathy becomes worse. When a
glomerular capillary thickens, kidney disease develops in time,
whereas muscle is a tissue that can form new capillaries readily.
Therefore, the thickness of capillaries in a muscle may not progress
to clinical capillary disease, so that there may be an entirely
different capillary turnover rate in different tissues.

DR. LEVINE: How do you view the Vracko theory that the capillary thickenings are not the result of increased production of
collagen-like material, but represents a remnant of dead cells
superimposed one upon another.

DR. KNOWLES: I will continue on two things that Roger started.
The really different aspects of the studies were that in the view
of Siperstein there was a much higher prevalence of basement membrane thickening in the pre-diabetic, and secondly, Siperstein's
data did not relate closely to age of the patient or duration of the
disease. On the other hand, Williamson's findings show that with
age the membranes get thicker in both normals and diabetics. The
crux of the matter is whether the slopes of the curves are different.

In Williamson's data the thickening increased more rapidly with
age in diabetic men only in comparison with non-diabetic men. The
rate of increase in diabetic women was not different from that of
non-diabetic women.

DR. SPRITZ: I don't think there is any argument on the part
of anyone that diabetes thickens basement membranes. So that even
if the diabetic curves were steeper, that does not get to the
basis of the argument that we are trying to resolve.

DR. KNOWLES: Well, yes it does! Roger raised the crucial
question of control and the disease. The St. Louis group would
like to relate control to the vessel thickness. Williamson's
group examined diabetics and normals and extrapolated the figures
back to age ten. From these data one can say that the pre-diabetic
person has normal basement membrane thickening prior to his onset
of diabetes. But, I am dubious of the validity of extrapolation
because of the curvilinearity of the regressions.

Another point which has arisen in this argument relates to
the methods used in fixation of the tissues. Siperstein uses osmic
acid and the Williamson group uses glutaraldehyde. Between people
who work in this field there is about a 50:50 division with regard
to their usage of these fixatives. The osmic acid method of fixation arose from the Rockefeller University group.

DR. ORCI: Indeed, osmic acid was the first fixative used in
electron microscopy. Today 99% of the workers prefix with glutaraldehyde, then postfix with osmic acid.

DR. KNOWLES: At a recent conference on membrane measurement,
some workers reported using osmic acid, while others used glutaraldehyde. These fixatives give a very different type of tissue to
look at. For all we know, diabetics and normals may respond differently when examined with these fixatives. Siperstein has emphasized this point in his arguments. As a matter of fact, he
published an article in the journal DIABETES about a year ago
(125) that when using Williamson's methods he got the same results
that Williamson got. So it may very well be that different fixatives are responsible for the differences in results.

There is another point on which I find myself in agreement
with Dr. Unger. This is with regard to the specificity of the
test in choosing whether or not to measure the thinner or the
thicker sections. I would have hoped that Williamson would have
taken his measurements both ways, measuring both the thick and the
thin section. In that manner we could see whether specificity
and sensitivity of the test could be established. I agree again,
it is very much like looking at the glucose tolerance test, look-

ing at both the high and the low responses.

DR. SPRITZ: There are discrepancies between basement membrane thickening and renal diabetic complications in a functional sense.

The chemical nature   DR. WOLF: Is the thickening collagen?
of the thickened
basement membrane   DR. ORCI: No, the thickening of base-
                              ment membrane is not due to collagen
fibers, but to a "biochemically" collagen-like material, at least in part.

DR. WOLF: It is just called collagenous. In other words, this is a bad term. If it is not collagen it should not be called collagenous. Is it an hydroxyproline? Because proline is part of the manufacturing process of collagen and elastin. Smooth muscle cells make collagen and elastin. Is there any evidence that pericytes are fundamentally smooth muscle cells?

DR. ORCI: There are immunochemical and ultrastructural evidence that they belong to the family of smooth muscle cells: for instance, they may contain a large number of contractile filaments.

DR. LEVINE: Lelio, you said something before about it not being collagen but it is approaching collagen, right? Since it contains 8% to 12% hydroxyproline, and it contains a certain percentage of hydroxylysine, it might be classified among the collagens. So, therefore, what is wrong with calling it collagen? Is it because it does not have the same periodicity as collagen?

DR. ORCI: Yes, from a morphological point of view.

DR. WILLIAMS: To quote from Vracko: "There is a lamina that is a layer of extracellular material of relatively uniform thickness composed principally of collagen-like protein and glycoprotein which normally forms an interface between parenchymal cells and connective tissue." (141)

DR. LEVINE: Well, he has every right as an electronmicroscopist to think that it is not collagen because it does not look like it, but it belongs to the collagen group, chemically.

DR. CAHILL: I referred earlier to Danish work currently in
                              progress that shows that you cannot
Kidney Lesions   detect any severe abnormality in the
                              kidney by biopsy early in the juvenile
diabetic, but four to five or more years later you begin to see it, particularly if control has been poor. The most recent data that show the kidney can be altered quite easily in the experi-

mental diabetic animal were collected by Mauer in the Minneapolis group (84). All of you may have heard that Mauer and Michaels of Minneapolis made a rat streptozotocin-diabetic, and within a period of six months there was a mesangial accumulation that looked like early diffuse glomerulitis. They took the diabetic kidney and transplanted it into an isogenetic non-diabetic and then during the next few months some of the lesions actually reversed themselves! This supports the contention that at least the kidney changes are responsive to the decreased insulin - high glucose abnormality.

DR. SPRITZ: I would like to offer the suggestion that the possibility of decreased insulin action could produce long term tissue changes by other than osmotic effects or hyperglycemia.

DR. KNOWLES: Considering some of Hansen's observations, and looking at her specimens, it is difficult for me to detect a difference between these diabetic kidneys and those of normal aging without controls. One cannot biopsy people year after year in order just to obtain simple data.

DR. CAHILL: The patients being followed in Lundbaek's clinic by Hansen et al. showed no abnormal changes in the first few years. However, after three or four years of diabetes significant structural changes were seen, so there is no question in my mind that the abnormality is a sequela of the diabetes. But the problem remains: do the changes represent an age factor only or an age factor plus diabetes? To my knowledge the Danish group has not studied normal controls. You simply cannot do that. Therefore you must rely on the evidence of normal kidney histology in aging non-diabetics as compared to abnormalities found in diabetic patients during the first two years of the onset of the diabetes.

DR. KNOWLES: There are two things regarding Mauer's work that I would like to comment on. First, what is the nature of the accumulated material that they found in alloxanized rats? I have talked with pathologists interested in nephrology and diabetes, and they are not certain that this is related to the diabetes. The second point is that you must have data beyond the abstract of their work since the definitive work has not yet been published. The study is of great interest, however.

DR. CAHILL: What Mauer, Michaels and this whole group has shown is that in this mesangial area of the capillary loops of the glomeruli there is an accumulation of stainable material which contains several immunoglobulins and this is how they found this out. The function of the mesangium is like that of the reticulo-endothelial system. It is a macrophage that picks up odds and ends and may metabolize some and serves as a sort of garbage cleaning maneu-

ver inside the kidney. But if you have a leak in the basement membrane, it saturates the tissue and exceeds the capacity of the mesangial cell to clean this up. Thus the accumulation.

DR. KNOWLES: Another of my objections is they did not seem to
have any controlled experiments showing rats who were alloxanized
and then treated with insulin.

DR. CAHILL: No, they did not do that but what they have done,
which is better than that, is to render rats diabetic with alloxan
or streptozotocin, in whom islets have been transplanted. They
then rendered those rats normal by transplanting islets from the
normal animals and the lesion did not develop. This is about the
most striking fundamental data on the kidney. Thus, the capacity
to transplant a rat kidney and keep it viable is a fantastic research tool in which you can study the effects of the environment.

DR. WILLIAMS: I would like to emphasize an important point
regarding dialysis. There are a great many deaths within about six
months after starting the dialysis procedure in uremic diabetics.
Of course, you do not have as a control undialyzed patients in the
same stage of uremia, but the incidence of death in that period of
six months was many times higher than it was in diabetics with
uremia in whom dialysis had not been started during the previous
six months.

DR. WOLF: While we are discussing the kidney would you fit
Najarian's work in with that? What
The fate of the   Najarian did in humans was to trans-
Transplanted kidney   plant kidney into diabetic humans in
the management of their glomerular
sclerosis and after four years there is still no evidence of glomerular sclerotic changes in the transplanted kidney (89).

DR. CAHILL: I don't think he or anyone else can say that.
There have been one or two hundred transplants into diabetics. In
the first place they don't biopsy them because they don't want to
bother them. In the second place, when the kidney undergoes immuno-
rejection it is totally impossible to tell whether or not there are
any diabetic changes because it is invaded so extensively by all
sorts of cells.

DR. SPRITZ: We had two pathologists from Montefiore go over
some of these diabetics who rejected kidney transplants, and the
rejection phenomena so dominated the picture that they could not
see the possibility of glomerular changes due to the diabetes.

DR. WOLF: I just called your attention to this because I
think it should be included in these proceedings so let me read

just one paragraph here. This is taken from Najarian. It reads,
"There has been no evidence of recurrent diabetic nephropathy in
the transplanted kidneys, ten one-year biopsies and six two-year
biopsies, and two three-year biopsies have been interpreted by an
independent pathology group as only showing mild rejection. There
was no evidence of diabetic nephropathy. Secondary complications
of diabetes contributing to renal failure, hypertension, and urin-
ary tract infection are problems that do not differ from that in
non-diabetic patients." (89) You would probably say that was
too short a time.

DR. CAHILL: Yes, according to the Danish workers it would
take two to five years before these changes would be evident.

DR. WILLIAMS: You also have to consider that all these people
have been literally plastered with glucosteroids which markedly
alter the fibroblasts, their metabolism, growth and so forth. So
it is not a comparable set-up.

DR. WOLF: One of the most tragic complications of diabetes –
indeed a major cause of blindness in
Retinopathy   the U.S. – is retinopathy. What do we
understand about its pathogenesis? Is
it really due to basement membrane thickening as in the case of the
kidney, or is the nature of the vascular lesion different?

DR. LEVINE: What is the difference between a pericyte in the
kidney and a mural cell in the retina?

DR. ORCI: The mural cell is really a pericyte and the mesangial cell is the equivalent of the pericyte also.

DR. LEVINE: We have been discussing the thickening of the
basement membrane in diabetes. Do equivalent changes actually occur
in the retina? I have not seen a demonstration of the thickening
of the basement membrane in the retina and neither have I under-
stood how this would lead to microaneurysms. Does the retinal
lesion at all have any relation to the lesion in the kidney?

DR. CAHILL: We really have no solid data on the eye and we
have too little comparative data. We don't really know whether
it is the same process as occurs in the other microvascular structures. There are at least two fairly distinct pathologic processes
in the retina of the diabetic: one is the macula edema, the maculopathy, and the other is the tendency for new vessel formation.
These two appear to be independent of each other; it is a paradox.
In some patients a severe maculopathy may progress to total legal
blindness. Others are blinded by diabetic retinopathy. They get
new vessels and fronds. Leaking occurs for reasons no one has

explained as far as I know. This kind of new vessel formation with
its associated bleeding can be treated by reducing the vascular
need of the rest of the eyeball. Now, how on earth these little
vessels know it is time to stop growing, so there is a reduction
in the total metabolic mass in the rest of the eye remains to be
explained but may reflect the influence of a humeral substance
akin to nerve growth-factor and tumor angiogenesis-factor that may
be very similar. As there is some factor that malignant tumors
produce that make benign vessels grow into the tumor, or any kind
of malignant tumors, there may be some abnormal signal that is
telling the capillary of the diabetic eye to proliferate and become leaky. How this correlates with total metabolic mass and how
it leads to blindness, and why these two occur in only 10% of the
patients who eventually get into major trouble, and the other 90%
do not, is a puzzle!

Pregnancy is hardest on the eye. When a diabetic of 15 to
20 years, gets pregnant she may develop retinitis proliferans and
then go on to total blindness, even including a hemorrhagic glau-
coma. We even had one or two situations where abortion was necessary to prevent blindness. Once the abortion takes place, the eye
disease seems to become quiescent. We don't know why this happens.

DR. WOLF: Aging has been referred to several times. I think
it is of interest that in the retina, the maculopathy or macular
degeneration, is a feature of aging that occurs independently of
diabetes and it also occurs in diabetes. But the small blood vessel growth is not a feature of aging, so these two in this respect
are quite distinct. Just as a side comment, Dr. Bernard Haber who
works at our Institute in Galveston, has grown glial cells in culture, together with capillaries. He has been able to demonstrate
the capillary-trophic factor in this preparation and is now in the
process of recovering and doing an aminoacid analysis of these
substances (61).   It would be interesting to see, as you point
out, to what extent this is similar or identical or grossly related
to these other trophic chemicals.

DR. CAHILL: The nerve growth-factor, the tumor angiogenesis-
factor, and the epidermal growth-factor are all of great potential
interest. We know that Choah Ho Li's pituitary factor that mobil-
izes adipose tissue free fatty acids, is a modified growth hormone
a ACTH. All of these probably have homologies in amino acid sequences, areas that are insulin sensitive and areas that are glucagon sensitive. Perhaps hypophysectomy for diabetic retinopathy
may have been a little helpful after all. In a randomized double-
blind group the incidence of remission, or at least postponement,
of progression ran about 50% to 60% as against the incidence of
spontaneous remission of retinopathy, which is in the order usually
of 10 to 20 per cent. But looking at it objectively with all the

morbidity that accompanied the hypophysectomy, severe hypoglycemic
reactions, the transient diabetes insipidus, and finally the re-
crudescence of retinopathy one or two years later, the whole thing
was not really worth it. Also, tragically, some of the patients
who had the best demonstration of total hypophysectomy by developing thyroid insufficiency and complete adrenal insufficiency, and
no detectable growth hormone, even after arginine stimulation of
hypoglycemia, went away with "galloping" retinopathy anyway.

DR. WOLF: In a very interesting article, Najarian has reported the subsidence of the retinal change in individuals who had
had renal transplants (90).   Why is it that the retinal changes
subside to a substantial extent following renal transplantation?

DR. KNOWLES: I think it is going to take a lot more clinical
observation of renal transplants in regard to their survival in
the diabetic and change in the retina.

DR. WOLF: Dr. Spritz, will you please discuss the neuropathy
of diabetes?

Neuropathy

DR. SPRITZ: We are trying to find a
system in which tissue dysfunction, a complication of diabetes, can
be studied in an experimental setting. In this effort, many of us
were stimulated by Spiro's work, in which he shows bridges between
the insulin deficient experimental diabetic animal, and the possible
production of abnormal tissue (130).   We have focussed on the
peripheral nerve in experimental diabetic animals.

A specific dysfunction that can be induced in animals made
deficient in insulin is alteration in conduction velocity in nerves.
This has been demonstrated in rats, within several weeks after the
induction of experimental diabetes. Nerve conduction velocity decreases also in human aging and in human diabetes.

There is evidence that in man neuropathy may be corrected in
part with insulin administration. We rendered rats and rabbits
diabetic with streptozotocin or alloxan and examined the peripheral
nerve. Since the Schwann cell itself wraps around the nerve fiber
and provides the myelin, any abnormalities we can show probably
represent dysfunction of the Schwann cell.

Fig. XXXV shows some of the evidence in man that in human
diabetics, the loss of myelin follows a segmental pattern where
the area serviced by one Schwann cell ends and the next one begins.
A decrease in myelinization would suggest a dysfunction of individual cells. This appears to be what happens early in the disease.
Later the nerve fibers themselves become involved (Fig. XXXVI).
Diabetic neuropathy is, therefore, much more than a disease of

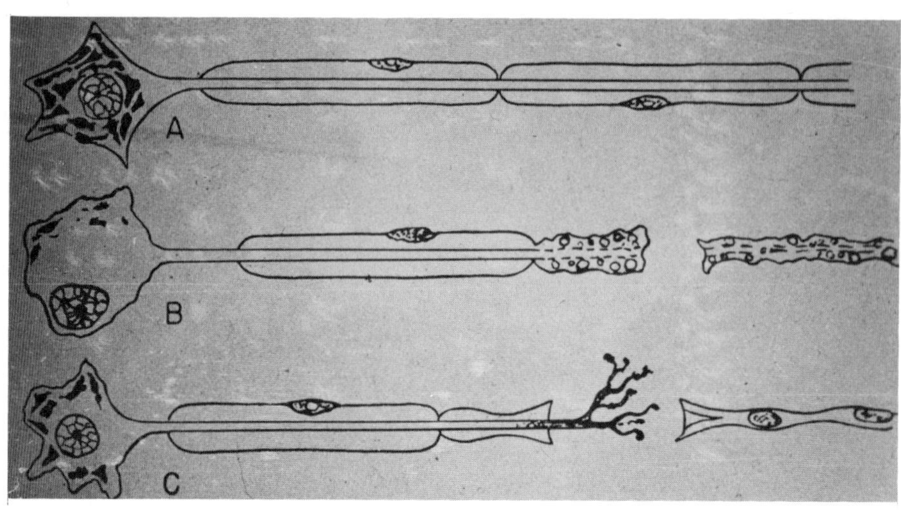

FIG. XXXV. Diagrammatic representation of segmental loss of myelin
in experimental diabetes. A- normal nerve. B - segmental myelin
degeneration. C - fragmentation of axon.

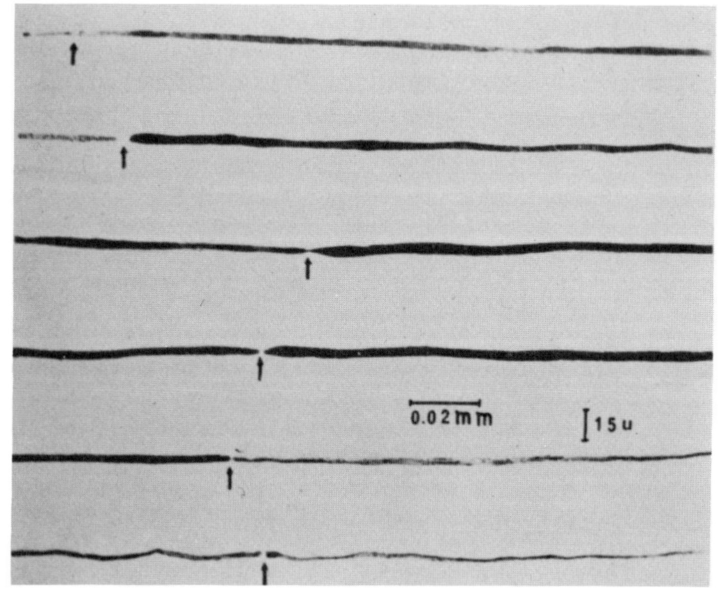

FIG XXXVI. Part of a single nerve fibre from a diabetic with neuropathy illustrating internodes of almost similar length, but variable
in diameter (osmium tetroxide).

myelin since nonmyelinated fibers are also affected by the disease.

We have made observations on nerves removed at autopsy from humans of different ages and found a myelin loss that correlated fairly well with age. We have seen a similar lesion appearing in the course of experimental diabetes in animals. Associated with the loss of myelin there was a decrease in conduction velocity. There was some indication that insulin could mitigate the process but the work is still preliminary and therefore the inference is uncertain. We are now attempting to identify the metabolic process whereby the Schwann cell fails to keep up with the job of myelin production. The relatively prompt occurrence of decreased nerve conduction in the experimentally diabetic animals makes it unlikely that the vasa vasorum are at fault. There are hints that the polyol mechanism described earlier may be implicated but it is too early to say.

DR. WOLF: Can you tell us about the vasa vasorum and the vasa nervorum of peripheral nerves in aging people and in nonogenerians, and in relation to a comparable degree, in diabetics, or any other person? Is there any relationship?

DR. CAHILL: I do not think that there are any good data. In fact, most of the neuropathies, when you begin talking to the neurologists, particularly with regard to the mononeuropathies, are felt to be vascular.

DR. KNOWLES: Where do you fit in the autonomics, bladder, etc?

DR. CAHILL: I don't know. The bladder may be just part of the metabolic abnormality.

DR. WOLF: Dr. Levine, what can you tell us about the occurrence of vascular lesions after the removal of the pancreas?

Experimental and Natural Models – Effects of Pancreatectomy on Macro- and Neuro-vascular Lesions

DR. LEVINE: As far as we know pancreatectomy is not followed either by microvascular disease or by hastening of atherosclerosis in the species that have been studied. An example is the dog. Ricketts studied a genetically pure bred strain of beagles. He performed pancreatectomies and treated a group strictly according to the Joslin criteria; some were treated poorly according to these criteria and he had normal controls. Atherosclerosis if anything, was a little less evident in the depancreatized group even when inadequately treated. There certainly was not a worsening of the situation. I also want to remind you, and this is something we should come back to, that

there is good evidence that hypercholesterolemia and deposition of
cholesterol in arteries in such animals as the rabbit seems to be
delayed by pancreatectomy and promoted by insulin. This is a very
important point in relation to large blood vessel disease in certain diabetics. Large blood vessel disease is not found directly
related to pancreatectomy.

There were a series of human pancreatectomies studied at the
Mayo Clinic in which very mild, beginning retinal changes were
found in one or two individuals (17). There are other series in
which the retinal changes were more progressive and closely resem-
bled socalled familial juvenile diabetes. The pathological changes
are convincing but the quantitative relation -- that is the number
of patients involved -- who had microvascular disease, was rather
small (25). Those who do not like to think of pancreatectomy
followed by microvascular disease will argue that when you find it,
it happens to be a pancreatectomy in an individual with genetic
tendencies. And those who argue the other way will say, "Yes, you
see there are changes even after a pancreatectomy." Dogmatic evidence for either point of view is just not present.

DR. SPRITZ: We have observed neuropathy in certain experimental animals with insulin-deficient types of diabetes. Within
six months or a year after pancreatectomy nerve conduction velocity
is decreased and we have some evidence that indicate a disturbance
in certain aspects of metabolism of nerves.

DR. WOLF: Can you demonstrate microvascular lesions in these
cases?

DR. SPRITZ: Not in the animals. In man, there are at least
two kinds of neuropathies. One is a symmetrical, chronic, progressive disorder involving vibratory sense and other posterior
column functions that are probably not related to vascular abnormality. The type that involves the vasa vasorum hits the whole
nerve and knocks out all of its functions, the so-called mononeuropathies.

DR. WILLIAMS: Total pancreatectomy is a poor model of human
diabetes because you always get extensive nutritional and metabolic
changes beyond those associated with diabetes; you are not only
removing insulin but glucagon. You are also impairing the function
of secretin, pancreozymin, gastrin, serotonin and other substances.

DR. KNOWLES: There are several cases of depancreatized persons living 25 to 30 years. One in LANCET about eight years ago
(145) and another in one of the German journals where nothing
happened to the patients (71).

DR. LEVINE: Coming to the humans, there is the famous contrast between two series of patients with pancreatic fibrosis associated with hemochromatosis: the series

Hemochromatosis and
Hepatic Effects

in Boston and the series in Cleveland. The series in Cleveland had small vessel disease but the series in Boston did not (6).

DR. KNOWLES: Five or six years ago, we saw about 35 cases of hemochromatosis and studied their kidneys extensively (69). We could never find significant kidney pathology although about two-thirds of them had had known hyperglycemia in life. We matched this series with a control group of Laennec's nutritional cirrhosis and then with a diabetic group. Then we re-examined the sections blindly and in randomized fashion. But we could never find the nodules of Kimmelstiel-Wilson's disease. We had some thick membranes, but they were no different from the thick membranes of the cirrhotic group. We thought they coincided somewhat with Bloodworth's findings of cirrhotic glomerulosclerosis (110). And that is as far as we got.

DR. WILLIAMS: Well there is one thing that bothers me about the study of hemochromatosis. There are apt to be disturbances of multiple organs: the liver, adrenals or others. Iron metabolism is greatly disturbed. We know that as you change the ratio of these different metals, you can change the function of a large number of enzymes. We do not know the extent to which these higher levels of iron will displace or otherwise interfere with the important functions of magnesium, calcium, and quite a number of other components.

Chapter VI - MACROVASCULAR DISEASE - ATHEROSCLEROSIS

DR. LEVINE: While small vessel disease seems to be specifi-
cally related to diabetes, what about large vessel disease, atherosclerosis? Suppose I were to postulate that insulin is really the
villain in this story. We know that insulin promotes lipid formation, could it induce greater activity of the myointimal cell within
the blood vessels, and therefore result in more atherosclerosis?
I would say that there is fairly good evidence that the adult-onset
diabetic with minimal hyperglycemia but with relatively high insulin and high fat is the one that has most of the atherosclerosis.
We never seem to see a case of gangrene in a juvenile diabetic.

DR. CAHILL: I would like to argue a little against that.
Perhaps juveniles do not live long enough to manifest atherosclerosis, whereas obese people are often long-lived and are known to
have three or more times the basal amount of insulin. Nevertheless
obesity is not highly correlated with atherosclerosis.

DR. WILLIAMS: Considering a large number of obese patients
in the 45 year age group, half of whom are diabetic, we know that
the obese non-diabetic has a higher insulin level than the diabetic
obese person but does not seem to have a higher incidence of atherosclerosis or infarction. Furthermore, there is not a great increase
in gangrene in obese non-diabetics.

DR. LEVINE: In diabetics insulin is acting on a basic genetic
                        dysplasia which affects fibroblasts
The vascular effects   derived from myocells. This has no-
of insulin lack or   thing to do with the blood sugar or
insulin excess   lipids. The non-diabetic patients do
                        not seem to have this genetic dysplasia.
Therefore excessive amounts of insulin may not accentuate the development of atherosclerosis.

DR. CAHILL: One cannot argue against that.

DR. LEVINE: But you know Duff in his studies demonstrated
in rabbits that insulin increased the severity of atherosclerosis
(31). Stamler did the same thing in chickens (131). The reason
I want to avoid sounding dogmatic about this is that maybe
we are taking a very large portion of our diabetic patients and
really not doing them any good by administering the kind of treatment which encourages greater insulin activity. I would like to
go back perhaps to the old, old treatment of keeping everyone almost fasting, and reducing not only the degree of hyperglycemia,
but also the degree of atherosclerosis instead of giving them
drugs or insulin.

DR. WILLIAMS: Major atherosclerotic changes develop much earlier in the life of diabetics than in nondiabetics. They are the main cause of death with over 60% of diabetics dying of coronary disease. In addition there is increased frequency of cerebrovascular disorders, gangrene, and arterial disturbances in other parts of the body. Deficient insulin action leads to a large variety of alterations in lipids, glycoproteins, collagens, and very likely in the smooth muscle cells, which play an important role in the pathogenesis of atherosclerosis (143).

DR. LEVINE: Macroangiopathy and atherosclerosis seem to me to be more the result of insulin _excess_ than of insulin lack! The reason I say this is as follows: the adult-onset diabetic who has arteriosclerosis in the limbs and threatening gangrene, is generally a person with higher blood levels of insulin than the juvenile diabetic. He may have absolutely excessive amounts at least for long periods, and a very mild diabetes. Yet he gets the worst type of large blood vessel disease. Secondly, while it is true that lipoprotein lipase activity depends to a certain extent on the presence of insulin, I am not at all sure that lipoprotein-lipase deficiency would lead in any way to atherosclerosis. The worst deficiency of lipoprotein lipase is in chylomicronemia, and chylomicronemia by itself generally does not lead to atherosclerosis. Thirdly, insulin is definitely associated, together with glucose, in promoting the formation of lipids in the liver and in the production of lipoproteins in high amounts. The other reason that I favor this view is the fact that during World War I and World War II, loss of weight and loss of lipid by the body as a whole was associated with the lack of overt glycosuric diabetes. At the same time there was a great diminution, or almost a complete absence, of large vessel disease in those areas of the world which were nutritionally deficient during the Wars.

The adult diabetics of Japan until recent years had very little gangrene (53). I visited the Osaka Clinic in 1963 and they had one case of gangrene in the whole of Southern Japan in studies covering a 15-year period. And yet they had a large number of diabetics. On the other hand, Japanese who live in Hawaii and California show a great degree of atherosclerosis. The diet of the Japanese in Japan has always been very high in carbohydrate and also, as we all know, very high in sodium chloride. However, their carbohydrate was mainly in the form of starch. In the areas of the world where carbohydrate consumption is mainly in the form of sucrose, the lipoprotein levels, the triglyceride levels and the degree of atherosclerosis seem to be greater. There is enough epidemiological evidence to cast suspicion on sucrose and to suspect insulin as a promoter of atherosclerosis rather than its preventer (134).

DR. WILLIAMS: May I make a comment or two? It has been definitely shown in rats that if you inject
The importance   insulin in large doses over a period
of obesity   of weeks you can cause some changes of
                                atherosclerosis. However you would find
more coronary disease among 45 year old diabetic women weighing
approximately 250 pounds, than among similarly obese non-diabetic
women. Both groups will have a hypernormal production of insulin,
particularly after glucose, but the level of insulin in the non-
diabetic group will be distinctly higher than in the diabetics.
Yet, the incidence of cardiovascular disorders is much higher in
the diabetic than in the non-diabetic.

DR. LEVINE: Would you say that if you took this 45 year old
diabetic group, that is the mild, obese diabetic female, and reduced their body weight that you would decrease the production of
insulin, and also that if you could keep them reduced you would
decrease the incidence of atherosclerosis as well?

DR. WILLIAMS: I would say that if you were able to reduce them
you would decrease the amount of hyperglycemia; you would also decrease the plasma levels of immunoreactive insulin and you would
increase the number of insulin receptors, and I think that you
would also decrease the chances of atherosclerosis.

DR. LEVINE: I concede that your argument concerning the 45
year old group is indeed a potent one. However, the reason I am
trying to champion the other point of view is this: I think that
we are not going to reduce the amount of coronary disease or the
number of attacks and the amount of gangrene, etc., until we im-
press upon the mild diabetic who has the tendency to hyperinsulinism
that the way he should be treated must be by weight reduction,
thereby reducing the insulin by diet, and by avoiding exogenous
insulin at all, nor should he be given materials which would induce
more insulin secretion.

DR. WILLIAMS: Instead of talking to him about reducing the
insulin, I would emphasize the importance of the reduction of weight.

DR. LEVINE: I agree.

DR. WOLF: You will recall that at one time it was thought that
the mechanism responsible for the adult onset diabetes was arteriosclerosis which affected the pancreas, therefore that the large
vessel disease was primary and insulin deficiency secondary to the
vascular lesions.

DR. LEVINE: At this point I should like to hear from the
lipid expert in the group.

DR. SPRITZ: I would like to talk about the relationship of
diabetes to hypertriglyceridemia and then come back to the issue of
the role of lipids and insulin in athero-
Lipoproteins and   sclerosis. If we accept that hyperlipi-
Macrovascular Disease   demia and both hypercholesterolemia and
hypertriglyceridemia constitute real
risk factors for vascular disease, the question is whether the risk
to the diabetic patient, with regard to vascular disease, operates
through this mechanism or not. Perhaps it is independent of this
mechanism or, more likely, risk relates both independently to the
diabetes as well as to the lipids.

There are not a great number of studies in which the total display of lipid concentrations in diabetics have been observed. One
of these was that of Ed Bierman and Marie New done at the New York
Hospital some years ago (92). I think that they came to one conclusion: most diabetics of all ages matched against people of similar age, seemed to fall within the normal range for both cholesterol
and triglyceride although the mean is distinctly higher for triglycerides in the diabetic group than in the population in general.
However, if you look at it from another point of view, that is if
you are in a Center studying lipids, you will find that most patients
with hypertriglyceridemia also have abnormal carbohydrate metabolism.
But again, if you start with a population that is identified as
having diabetes, they do not really have markedly altered lipid
concentrations, and as a matter of fact such a study revealed that
cholesterol concentrations of the diabetics were really not different from those of their age-matched controls. Others have found
the same thing. In a hospital-based population you start with diabetics who have vascular diseases. I think that both Dr. Williams
and Dr. Levine are correct in arguing that there is a mechanism for
hypertriglyceridemia (which is really VLDL excess) in both insulin
depletion and insulin excess, either of which can produce hypertriglyceridemia. The cleanest cut amongst the insulin deficient
patients are the ones described by Dr. Bierman in Seattle: diabetics
with lipemia who seem to be a very special sub-set of the diabetic
population (5).   They have very high levels of triglyceride and
seem to have a defect of lipoprotein lipase. Their hypertriglyceridemia seems to get better with the administration of insulin and
concomitantly the lipoprotein lipase activity improves. The larger
group is probably the adult group who tend to have fasting hyperinsulinemia, obesity, and hypertriglyceridemia. Several people have
identified these patients as over-producers of very low density
lipoprotein (VLDL) and this is probably one of the bases for their
hypertriglyceridemia. They do not seem to have a defect in the
removal of triglycerides.

In a way that is the easy part of the problem. However, relating this to atherosclerosis is more uncertain. I think it has

been pretty clear for a long time that microvascular disease has
no relationship to plasma lipids, but macrovascular disease does.
However, the diabetic patient has an increased risk of developing
vascular disease at normal lipid concentration. My own tendency
would be to favor Dr. Levine's view. In general the higher levels
of pre-beta lipoproteins (that is the high VLDL) are found in the
patients we studied who have higher plasma insulin levels. These
are the ones in whom Reaven and others gathered evidence indicating
a true relationship between fasting insulin concentrations and triglyceride levels (112). There is another group of patients who
demonstrate this association between VLDL and hyperinsulinemia with
insulin resistance, the uremic patients on dialysis who almost all
have hypertriglyceridemia associated with high insulin levels. A
recent paper showed that patients with chronic uremia do have increased vascular disease (78). So I think we can conclude that
the hyperinsulinemic diabetic is susceptible to large vessel disease.

DR. LEVINE: I should like to remind you of an older experiment by Duff from McGill, who did some classical cholesterol feeding
of rabbits to produce atherosclerosis (31). When alloxan became
available he wanted to see if diabetes would aggravate the artificially induced atherosclerosis, in other words whether he would
worsen the degree of atherosclerosis. He made rabbits alloxan diabetic and then fed them the standard hypercholesterolemic diet.
Surprisingly, they developed much less atherosclerosis. When these
animals were given insulin, the degree of atherosclerosis became
more pronounced.

DR. WILLIAMS: Well, I like my human model better.

DR. LEVINE: Human models are indeed fine, yet nature is quite
uniform in its biochemical machinery and what one learns about a
bacterium one day is true (more or less) for the human by the next
week.

DR. WILLIAMS: What we have to reckon with also is the immuno-
assayable insulin. We know that obese diabetic patients have hyperglycemia but what is the evidence of excessive insulin action outside of its effect on fat tissue?

DR. SPRITZ: That is a very important point. The theory that
the insulin-resistant patient has hyperinsulinism because of that
resistance postulates that there are certain tissues not resistant
to insulin which are bathed by an excess of this insulin. As far
as I know, this is pure theory and there is no real evidence for
it. The hypothesis relating hyperinsulinemia to hypertriglyceridemia includes the fact that triglyceride or VLDL production is en-
hanced by the excess insulin. This could make it a function related

to insulin in which resistance is selectively absent. Hyperlipidemia in rabbits is so different from that in man as to make all
comparisons difficult.

DR. LEVINE: You mean that animals are different from people?
Yes, not everybody is equal but some are a little more equal than
others. Suppose we take the Carneau pigeon, is that good?

DR. SPRITZ: That is better, and let me say why I think it is
better. The rabbit makes cholesterol, stores great quantities of
lipid and then makes lipoproteins that do not exist in humans.
Further the rabbit is very susceptible to the effects of alloxan
with a degree of hypertriglyceridemia not found in human diabetics.

DR. LEVINE: The insulin story in promoting atherosclerosis
was repeated by Stamler in the omnivorous ("more human") chicken
(131).

DR. WOLF: Well, Norton, you will have to admit that it was
the rabbit that started the whole business of the great cholesterol
scare.

DR. SPRITZ: Well, assuming that was a good step, I would say
that it was really a lucky one.

DR. LEVINE: What would you say about Stamler's chickens?

DR. SPRITZ: Well, chickens have some beta lipoprotein -- more
than rabbits -- so they are more appropriate animals to study.

DR. LEVINE: They are omnivorous, they are not strictly herbi-
vorous animals and they get lesions resembling the human. Insulin
makes these lesions more extensive.

DR. KNOWLES: I have some data on macroangiopathies in juvenile diabetes.

DR. WILLIAMS: What is that based on? Everyone over the age
of three has some degree of atherosclerosis.

DR. KNOWLES: The presence of atherosclerosis is based on clinical myocardial infarction or angina and three cases with plaques
in the iliac artery requiring by-pass surgery. I call these symptomatic macroatherosclerotic obstructions. At autopsy every single
one of my juvenile diabetics has had severe coronary artery disease.
The average age of these would be in their 40s. The other thing
that is interesting about macroangiopathy in the juvenile diabetic
is the seriousness of the event. The diabetic with a myocardial
infarct survives on the average less than five years, according to

Joslin Clinic figures. In the juvenile population, survival time
was two or three years, and I have no patients that have lived
three years after the occurrence of a clinical symptomatic coronary
event. Also, we have a lot of "silent" infarcts without symptoms
that show up only on autopsy.

DR. WOLF. Did you say that autopsies on individuals who did
not die of coronary artery disease nevertheless showed massive
atheromatous involvement of the large blood vessels?

DR. KNOWLES: Absolutely. I have had one with one half of the
right ventricle virtually infarcted away with vascular calcium who
had no symptoms of coronary disease. This is a new field of vascular disease.

DR. LEVINE: And why not in the vessels of the lower limb?
What is the reason?

DR. KNOWLES: I asked Danowski about this, and he had not seen
peripheral occlusive disease. I have also asked Dr. Priscilla
White and she says it is rare. I will probably see it one of these
days, but I think it will be diffuse internal thickening rather
than distinct occlusion.

DR. WILLIAMS: There are differences even in the chemistry of
the atherosclerotic lesions that take place in the coronary arteries
compared with those in the aorta.

DR. CAHILL: I am not so sure that you would say that all these
occurrences in the arteries below the knees are spared in the juvenile diabetics. Although you may not get the terminal occlusion,
one sees severe, diffuse atherosclerosis and the evidence for this
is from the dialysis programs where A-V shunts result in loss of
fingers or even hands in diabetics.

DR. SPRITZ: I am not sure but that when the occlusive disease
occurs in the leg in young people that they can compensate for it
whereas when it occurs in older people then it leads to a more
malignant state.

DR. KNOWLES: Monkeberg's, not atherosclerosis, is the common
lesion. I think that an occlusion is unusual in Monkeberg's.
Thick toe nails and the shiny skin are the signs that go with occlusive vascular disease. This is very unusual, or at least it has
not occurred in my population. I think it is going to occur some
day because anything is possible.

DR. SPRITZ: There seem to be two types of diabetics who suffer myocardial infarctions at about the same age; that is, in their

40s. One group are the survivors of the microangiopathy period,
who then come to myocardial infarction after a long period of
insulin deficiency. The other group out of the blue, develop a
sudden myocardial infarction. The latter group have something
wrong with their carbohydrate metabolism but the two groups are
very different in every way.

DR. CAHILL: The second group have a high incidence of diabetic
relatives.

DR. SPRITZ: Yes, they do, and a high incidence of hyperlipidemia and they come to the same end point despite the difference in
their diabetes. One may also encounter myocardial infarction in
young people with abnormal glucose tolerance curves but normal
lipids. Therefore it appears that diabetes may contribute to coronary atherosclerosis independent of hyperlipidemia.

Chapter VII - THERAPY

     DR. WOLF: On the basis of the findings discussed in the last
couple of days, do you see a change in the customary canons for the
evaluation and management of diabetic patients?

     DR. KNOWLES: There might not be among those of us sitting at
this table, but I think in this country at large that there is a
change. This is based on what I hear at meetings and some of the
statements that have been made here today.

     DR. WOLF: I wonder if Roger would give a crisp response to
several questions:

What are the benefits of early detection of diabetes?

Suppose we could regulate the blood glucose within narrow
    limits, what would be achieved?

When is insulin required and, if so, what kind?

What is the place of oral hypoglycemics?

How does one select a diet?

What other drugs are potentially helpful and valuable
    in adult onset diabetes?

What are autonomic agonists and antagonists and what
    is the future of islet transplantation?

     DR. UNGER: You are asking me to do what a generation of out-
standing diabetologists have been unable to do! First, at the
present time we are in a very primitive stage, and we are just
beginning to get a good look at the basic questions. I mean, we
do not even really know much about what the human islets of Langerhans look like, what they appear like under electron microscopy
to people like Dr. Orci, and whether or not there will be a visible
lesion. I shall leave this meeting with a greater appreciation
of precisely how the islets of Langerhans function. I must admit
that I have never been an adherent of the strict diet control regimen. And yet, I cannot help but marvel at how the alpha-beta
cell couple permits a wide change in glucose turnover with minimal
change in glucose concentration. That is really one of their
primary functions. Why does nature keep the glucose concentration
within narrow range? There must be a good reason and it could be
to avoid the microangiopathy that afflicts those who cannot avoid
hyperglycemia.

DR. KNOWLES: Dr. F. M. Allen of Boston once said that a properly controlled diabetic would never develop any complications.
He published this about twenty years ago (3) and repeated the
statement again at the Atlantic City meeting about 15 years ago,
shortly before he died.

DR. UNGER: He reputedly said that a little hypoglycemia every
day was a prerequisite for good diabetic control. 98% of the diabetics that Dr. Marvin Siperstein looked at had basement membrane
thickening. One exception was a man whose diabetes extended back
to childhood, a matter of 22 to 23 years. He had been strictly
controlled on insulin and, indeed, had been hypoglycemic much of
the time. Physical examination revealed no evidence of eye ground
changes and there was no proteinuria. Since at Southwestern we are
more concerned about over-insulinization than we are about a little
glycosuria, we managed him rather loosely. Several years later
this patient was re-biopsied and, despite his loose control, there
was still no thickening of his basement membrane. I wonder whether
one well-studied case might not be better than a lot of statistical
information. I do not know how often other people are biopsied in
these other groups, and how often a patient with no history of pancreatitis and with a history of diabetes, can be found with normal
basement membranes. I think that the other questions Dr. Wolf
asked should be shared among all of us.

Islet
Transplantation

A question was asked about transplantation. I do not know if enough islets
can be made available to meet the needs
of the juvenile diabetic population.

DR. CAHILL: If you take a normal individual and lay his beta
cells out on a plane surface, he has approximately one square meter.
This is a crude calculation, but to grow enough beta cells for one
man would take hundreds of culture plates.

DR. KNOWLES: How many cells is that?

DR. CAHILL: One gram of cells.

DR. KNOWLES: How many islets are there in the human pancreas?
I heard that there were approximately one million.

DR. CAHILL: How many beta cells per islet? Would you say
that there are approximately five hundred?

DR. ORCI: No, there are more than that. In an islet 200
microns in diameter, there are roughly six thousand beta cells.

DR. KNOWLES: Is the suggested figure of 250,000 islets per

patient correct?

DR. ORCI: In the adult human pancreas, the number of islets
is estimated to range from 200,000 to 1,800,000.

DR. KNOWLES: I guess that would be based on normals, "Braaten's
transplants".   250,000 islets might be a minimum amount that would
work in man's pancreas.   Of course, if you went back to beta cells
the figures would be much higher.

DR. UNGER: How many diabetic children are there in the United
States?

DR. KNOWLES: There is about one juvenile diabetic in 1000
total population.   Since there are 200,000,000 people in the United
States, that means there would be approximately 200,000 juvenile
diabetics in the country today.

DR. CAHILL: Actually I think a couple of hundred thousand
is about right.

DR. KNOWLES: Coming back to the question, Stewart, that you
asked of Roger, I can see no evidence that what we have been doing
for the last decade or so has resulted
The value of strict con-   in any solid effect in changing the
trol of blood glucose   risk or the appearance of microangio-
                             pathy, or changing its course.   I
simply cannot see that any single event has altered this problem.
As far as returning the chemistry to normal, islet transplantation
may do it!   But as we see current diabetes treatment in this country, I am not sure that blood sugar can be returned to the normal
state.   And I do not think that there are any studies, at least
ones that satisfy me, to show that when we have returned blood
sugar towards normal, the course of the disease has been altered.
We can quote from studies the other way.   There are rare studies
which deal with grossly uncontrolled diabetes, according to everybody's standards and herein complications appear plentiful (33).
But I really cannot answer that question.

DR. KNOWLES: Table 3 summarizes data on juvenile diabetic
complications up to 1965.   At that time I took a summary of all
the studies on angiopathy in diabetics and rearranged the figures
so that the data were on cases where the diagnosis was made at 16
years of age or less and diabetes was known for ten years or more.
No matter where the cases came from (i.e., Joslin, Scandinavia,
all over), the prevalence of vascular disease was just overwhelm-
ing.   There is a point regarding duration which concerns the growth
spurt years and puberty.   If you subtract the number of years of
diabetes prior to puberty, the variance of the yearly developmental

Table 3. The Reported Prevalences of Complications (the findings are given as percentages of patients observed)

			No. Patients	Age at Diagnosis	Known Duration (YRS)	Retinopathy	Proteinuria	Calcification	Peripheral Vascular Disease	Hypertension	Cardiac Disease	Neuropathy	Cataracts
1	Eisle	1942	73	<15	20 →	42		30	3	20		10	16
	White	1948	220	<16	20 →	75	40	70		55	7		
	Wilson	1951	247	<30	10 →	64	25	67	3	19		6	2
	White	1956	1072		15–19	59	18	44		15			
	Immersland	1959	73	< 2	15–19	23	4.3	9		0			
	White	1960	478	<15	30 →	90	42	83+		43		48+	
	Dolger	1947	55	<20	5–22	100	44	11		42			
2	Chute	1948	47	<15	15 →		17	13		11	4	19	15
	Kerr	1952	63	<16	10 →	62	16	21			11	13	
	Collyer	1961	77	<16	10 →	90						52	31
	Grill	1948	105	<20	10 →		23						
	Fanconi	1948		<17	16		100						
	Pillow	1949	25	<15	20 →	51	40	28		28			4
	John	1949	52	<20	10 →	33							
3	Jackson	1949	75	<15	10 →	47	4	16		4	0		15
	Hardin	1956	140	<16	10 →	51							
	Martensson	1950	40	<20	9 →	35							13
	Sherrill	1951	14	<17	20 →	50	14			21			
	Daeschner	1951	41	<15	11 →	73	22			24			
	Grayzel	1951	24	<17	11 →	37	33	29					
	Guild	1952	40	<14	10 →	42	22	22		20		5	
4	Larsson	1952	33	<17	>15	72.8	30.3	14.3		33			
	Larsson	1962	153	<16	15 →	82	50	81		25	10		
	Lundbaek	1953	38	<20	15 →	84	18		3	50	3		5
	Engleson	1954	40	<21	10 →	90	87						
	Forsyth	1956	55	Child.	10 →	51	15			5	0		
	Joos	1957	44	<15	10 →	41	16			2		5	
	Danowski	1957	37	<10	10–19	19	54		0	16	0		
	Downie	1959	47	<21	20 →	41	26						
	Knowles	1965	78	<17	10 →	64	33	27		28		35	47

[1] Studies from the Joslin Clinic
[2] Studies from the Toronto Childrens Hospital, University of Toronto
[3] Studies from the University of Iowa
[4] Studies from Pediatric Clinic of the Crown Princess Lavisa Hospital, Stockholm, Sweden

rates of angiopathy becomes smaller. In this regard, Dr. Joseph
Williamson (65) came to the conclusion that basement membrane
thickening takes place after the growth spurt years. Does not
atherosclerosis start in the growth spurt years also?

DR. SPRITZ: Well, the plasma lipids change at about that time.

DR. KNOWLES: So it may be at the beginning of the growth spurt
years that changes take place in the vasculature of the diabetics,
of micro as well as macro angiopathies. The problem is an immense
one. All I can say is that if these vascular changes can be prevented by lowering blood sugars, we have not been very successful
in this country.

DR. SPRITZ: You keep saying "in this country". Is there
some evidence that this has been overcome in some other country?

DR. KNOWLES: I was just being polite. I had better say that
in my observation I have failed to detect any prevention of these
complications.

DR. WILLIAMS: Don't you think, Harvey, that you might be able
to achieve this goal in those in whom you are able to control the
blood sugar well?

DR. KNOWLES: I don't know, since no one has been able to control the blood sugar well. We had a panel at the American College
of Physicians meeting in New York on the subject of "brittle" diabetes. George Molnar of the Mayo Clinic, Robert Bradley of the
Joslin Clinic, Lester Baker from Pennsylvania and myself struggled
with the problem. We went right on down the line and tried to ar-
rive at a picture of what was the best we could do in the management of these difficult brittle juvenile diabetics. We could get
sugars coming down before meals, but we could not prevent post-
prandial rises. Fig. XXXVI describes a study that was done by
taking samples of blood sugar at any given moment, when the patients
were not expecting the test and they had no symptoms. The highest
asymptomatic level seen then was about 700. Our highest case now
was somewhere in the neighborhood of 1350, a patient with nephrosis.
We have evidence on "Why do they not have hyperosmolar coma?"

DR. CAHILL: Yes. You just caught him coming out of McDonalds!

DR. KNOWLES: Well, some of the blood sugars would stay up
there for about 48 hours. This was a good three-month project for
a fourth year medical student. When the sugars averaged between
600 and 700, the sodiums averaged around 130 so that tonicity was
not too high. We were able to show this in anephric diabetic patients before and after dialysis.

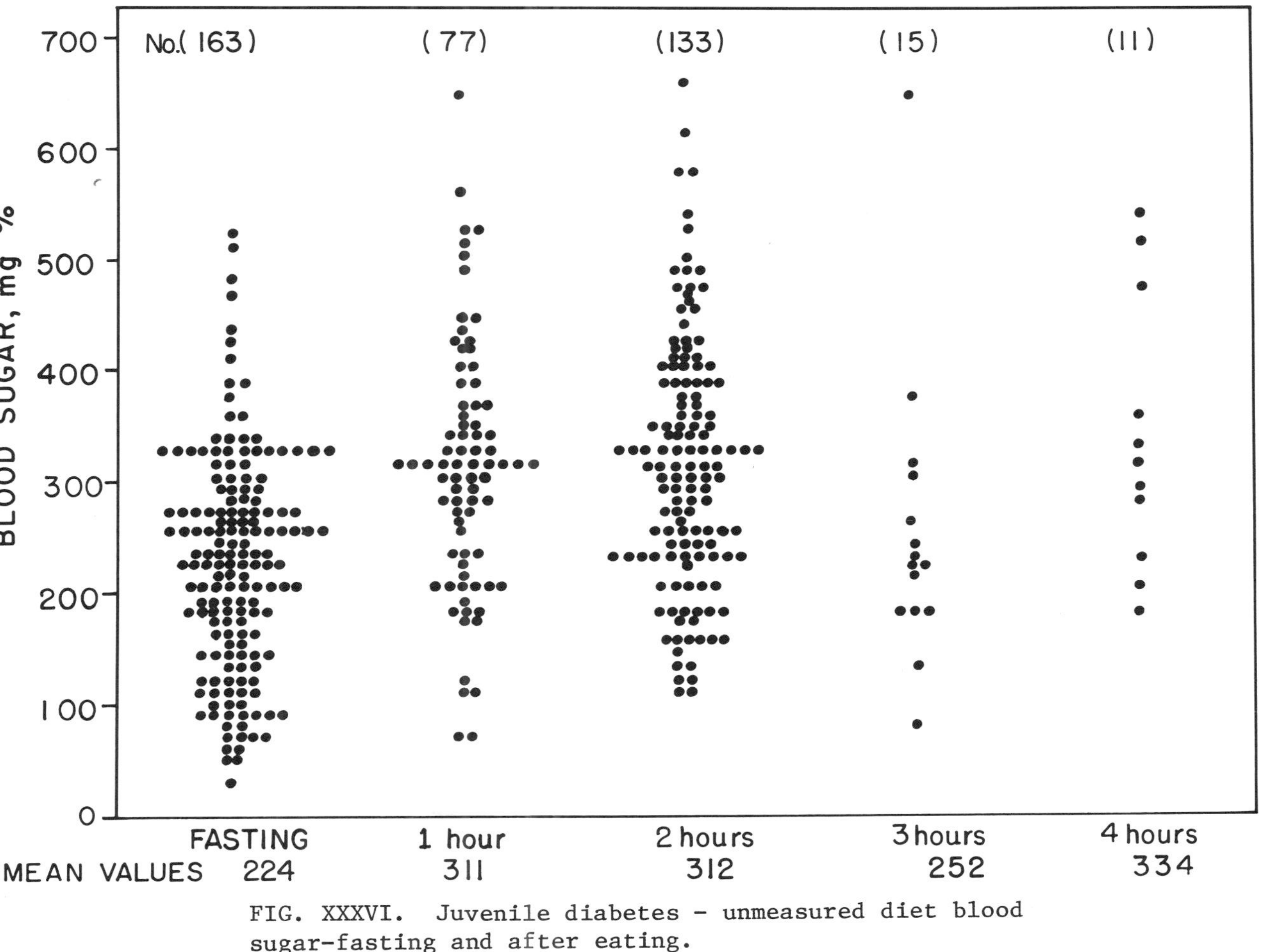

FIG. XXXVI. Juvenile diabetes – unmeasured diet blood sugar–fasting and after eating.

We found that the mortality rate in juvenile diabetes was not
quite as bad as we indicated during our discussions yesterday. It
was indicated that mortality was something on the order of 20% in
25 years cumulative mortality over time. This figure applies to
the 25th year. Mortality is the result of renal failure in 50 to
60 per cent of cases. Therefore, glomerulosclerosis is far and
away the major cause of death in the juvenile diabetic. Therefore
this business of control that Dr. Wolf just brought up could be of
considerable significance. Unfortunately, however, we do not seem
to be able to achieve it. Of course there may as well be significant influences of genetic and environmental factors with regard
to longevity and freedom from complications.

DR. UNGER: With regard to transplantation, even if it is
mathematically impractical, if a few patients can be controlled
successfully over a period of years just to determine the relationship of good control to compare it with vascular disease, it would
be worth the effort. I suspect that the mass studies will never
give us the answer.

DR. SPRITZ: I wonder what is the status now of the sensor
                                and the automated means of delivery
Implanted glucose   of insulin as studied through the use
regulatory devices   of electrodes.

DR. CAHILL: At the moment there are some three dozen of them
that are being studied. Soeldner and his colleagues are working
on the problem of the long term stability of the electrodes. There
are two general approaches. One, being used by Bessman, is glucose
oxidase as a solid state enzyme, which consumes oxygen with an adjacent oxygen electrode which measures oxygen changes, a function
of glucose concentration. We are working on a metal catalyst (by
"we" I mean Soeldner with engineers of the Space Science Corporation in Boston) which oxidizes glucose to gluconic acid. This is
a true glucose fuel cell and makes its own electric current directly.
It has been implanted in animals now for up to six months and still
maintains good fidelity; it has about a ten minute lag in its read-
out signal.

DR. LEVINE: Does it not develop tissue scarring with time?

DR. CAHILL: There is a degree of fibroplasia that develops
around it. We are trying now to test different anti-fibroplastic
polymers that would still allow free communication to glucose and
oxygen, and egress of gluconic acid. The engineers say that they
can make an electrode about the size of a 20-gauge needle that can
be inserted into a vascular or tissue space, but the biomedical
people caution us to stay out of the vascular space and have suggested that we stay in the extracellular fluid simply because any-

thing in the vascular space is much more likely to induce clotting.

DR. SPRITZ: That is surprising because when pacemakers are
implanted the tip is actually in the bloodstream.

DR. CAHILL: Yes, but only a small tip protrudes into the
bloodstream and scar tissue forms around it rather rapidly.

DR. SPRITZ: Yes, when you take them out you can see that scar
tissue has formed around, but they do protrude into the stream.
Many diabetics have them.

DR. LEVINE: May I ask a kind of pseudo-quantitative, or pseudo-
philosophical question in relation to blood sugar level and the
possible relationship to complications? Let us say we all agree,
whether we are adherents of strict or non-strict dietary control,
we do not want symptoms so that we will aim to have a minimal glycosuria, eliminate the problem of frequency, etc. Now, the next
question would be this. If, let us say as Roger puts it, the insulin-glucagon couple is very sensitive in maintaining a very narrow level of glycemia, that is, something in the order of 10 mg%
i.e., the usual normal, then if this is so, does any artificial
system need to keep it within such narrow limits? In other words,
I am asking the following: if we transgress and still keep the level
stable, according to our present standards, but not within the
limits of 10 mg%, is an extra 5 or 10 mg% so destructive that we
simply have to keep it precisely within this extremely narrow limit?
Because if that is so, then there is no point in quarreling now
with somebody whose blood sugar is 115 and another one that is 150
or 160, since we have to wait for artificially strict machinery
before we can do something. In other words, do we really have to
be as accurate as you think your couple is?

DR. UNGER: I really do not know. It may be a function of
time when you are talking about a five year old child. It may be
quite different for older cases.

DR. LEVINE: Right now there are some people who will collect
data and say that while they are not too convincing, they have
kept their diabetics at an average of 200, and here another group
of diabetics at 180, and shown that the group kept at 180 had less
complications than the one at 200. So, tell me what does that
mean?

DR. UNGER: I think those studies are meaningless.

DR. CAHILL: I was just going to say that since connective
tissue and their morphological changes have such long half-lives
of all the factors that we are measuring, mean hyperglycemic years

(like "Pack years" for smoking and carcinoma of the lung) is the
determinant.

DR. LEVINE: But is the years multiplied by a 10 mg. excess
equivalent to the years times 50 mg. excess?

DR. CAHILL: That is like asking if smoking three packs a day
for 10 years is equivalent to smoking one pack a day for 30 years.
Epidemiologically, there may be no difference but we simply do not
know the numbers exactly. Then, furthermore, there is probably a
tremendous variation in the population. There is the kid who has
an ambient glucose of 300 or 400 because he is a sloppy kid and
he takes his insulin every other day, and then tragically there is
the kid right next to him, who tests his urine four times a day
trying to do the best he can, gets the right diet, and yet both
of them go blind at age 25, and go on to uremia, and die. People
say, "Look, why bother to treat?"

DR. UNGER: It is clear that present day therapy does not prevent the microangiopathies and for that matter present therapy has
not prevented the hyperglycemia.

DR. KNOWLES: Well, George, I have never said that control
might not delay progression. If I ruled out control I would be
making a Type 2 error of experimental design, which I presume everyone in this room is familar with. I have seen no evidence that control does delay progression. In fact such control cannot be achieved
in this population.

DR. CAHILL: I am trying to get somebody to go back and study
the diabetics that we still see -- there
are probably no more than 30 or 50 of
Regular versus
long-acting insulin
them around -- who have been taking
insulin three or four times a day and
refused to go on the fancy new protamine zinc insulin that came out
in 1936, and the NPH in the 40s, and you get the impression that
these people have, indeed done better.

DR. LEVINE: Do such people have lesser swings?

DR. CAHILL: Probably.

DR. SPRITZ: Yes, Lukens has some of these data.

DR. KNOWLES: The best paper on that is R. D. Lawrence's on
92 cases (73). I have about 35 or 40 juvenile diabetics with
more than 30 years diabetes, and seven with more than 45 years.
Their diabetes has been managed with unmeasured diet. In this the
only complication that I have seen has been medial calcification

that appeared in the legs. But, unfortunately, these seven have
been on long-acting insulin all these years and they are all on
single dose regimens. Now, I ask the question: could it be that
after 30 years of treatment the risk of microangiopathies starts to
taper off? Could it also be that the people who escape microangiopathy are just the fortunate ones to have gone through that long
period and escaped, or who have been sorted out, or may be selected
out? Although the numbers are small, Fig. XXXVII shows that after
30 years, little microangiopathy seems to develop. A few developed
a few retinal aneurysms, but nothing else much happens. These are
the ones that become risks for macroangiopathies.

DR. CAHILL: You mean that once you lose the 50% that die of
nephropathy, the rest will suffer a coronary.

DR. WILLIAMS: What percentage of your juveniles have died
because of coronary heart disease?

DR. KNOWLES: I would guess not more than 15 to 20%.

DR. CAHILL: Oh, Harvey, no! Of all diabetics of the total
population that figure would be 70 to 80%, but for juvenile onset
it is about 20%.

DR. KNOWLES: But for juvenile-onset, it is only about 15 to
20%. Maybe the multiple shots saved some people. We have a fellow
who started insulin back in 1922, and he took four shots of regular
insulin a day, drinking a glass of orange juice every time he took
that shot. He died from simple cerebral thrombosis at age 80 after
some 40 years on this regimen. And he never had any other pathology
that we could determine in him. But his blood sugars were all over
the place.

DR. WOLF: What you are saying is, I think, that the 20% of the
individuals who make it through some 30 years without developing
retinopathy have a good chance of long life without serious complications.

DR. KNOWLES: Right, and if you read the Joslin data on the
victory medal group the results are quite striking, and the striking
thing is the absence of microangiopathies in those longstanding
diabetics (121).

DR. LEVINE: Is there not a possibility that this 20 to 25% is
just a different kettle of fish?

DR. KNOWLES: Sure. That's what I said a while back.

DR. LEVINE: But there is a marvelous description of retinopathy in a bunch of about 10 or 12 papers that appeared between

JUVENILE DIABETES - UNMEASURED DIET
RETINOPATHY
CUMULATIVE RISKS
80
70
60
50
40
30
20
10
0
% RISK
Retinopathy
Retinopathy (prevalence)
Neovascularization
Blindness
10
15
20
25
30
35
40
YEAR OF DIABETES

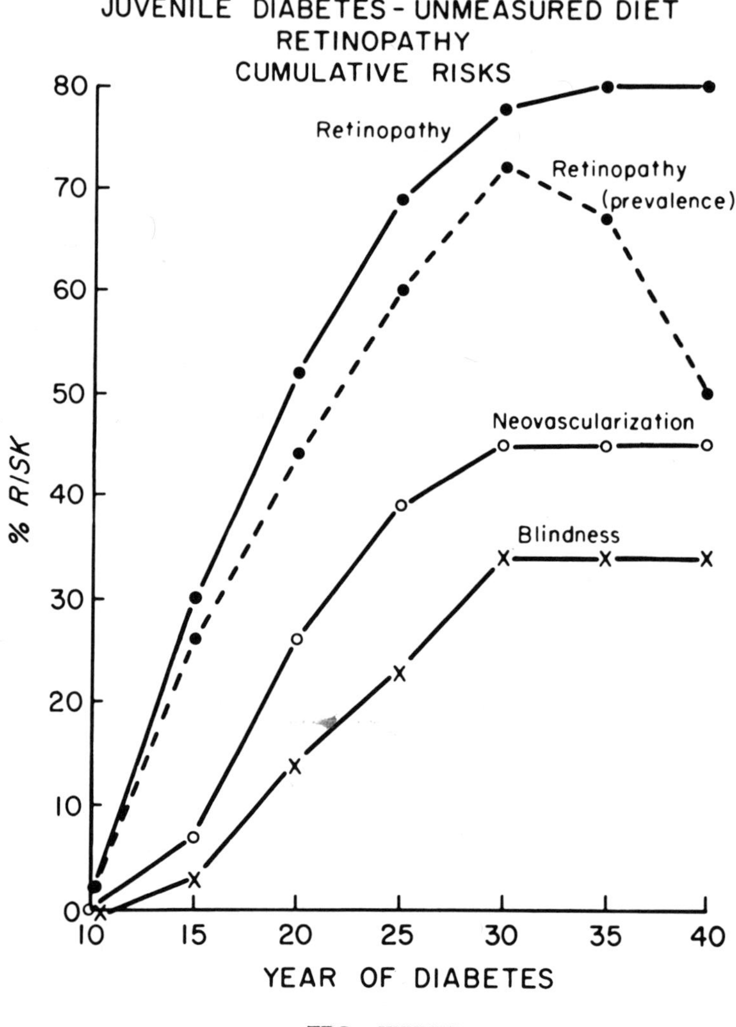

FIG. XXXVII

1870 and 1885 and they tell you neither about protamine zinc insulin
nor regular insulin, nor anything as being a determining factor.
These descriptions of retinopathy seem to have been rediscovered
in the 1930's. But you go back and look at those papers (those
drawings were absolutely fantastic) and they originated from the
immediate pupils of Mr. Helmholtz, the discoverer of the ophathal-
moscope (58).

DR. CAHILL: The point that I am getting at is this, was the
diabetic after 20 or 30 years or so of therapy, more at risk with
microangiopathy when he was on the single protamine zinc insulin
versus four doses per day of clear insulin. (Retrospectively,
those numbers could be determined). I am just saying that one
gets the impression in looking back, that the major wave of retinopathy developed in those cases that were seen in the late 1950's,
twenty years after the discovery of protamine zinc insulin.

DR. KNOWLES: Johnsson's paper is the one that backs this the
most and his figures are taken in Denmark, which covers the periods
wherein they had the two different insulins and on different regimens (64). It just depends on how people looked at these
things. In the 1930's we had an upswing of diabetic renal disease
at the Cincinnati General Hospital. That was the time we really
went to town in controlling diabetes because Dr. Lewis Owens,
now deceased, ran the Diabetes Clinic and he set up rigid schedules
which we followed. The reason that we had this upswing in diabetic
nephropathy was because he made us look for it for the first time.

DR. WOLF: Rachmiel, could I ask you to deal with the question,
                        "When is insulin required in the treat-
Indications for   ment of diabetes?"
Insulin therapy

DR. LEVINE: I think one would say insulin is required if insulin
is severely missing in a diabetic patient, and if not treated ketosis
might occur, or a degree of glycosuria which would lead to the
development of symptoms. Of course, I don't think you will get the
same answer from everybody, and this really depends on how tightly
you think one should control patients. Let me try to clear up one
thing: those of us who do not belong to a particular school and who
are a little bit more "loose", let us say, with blood sugar regulation and control, at least would like to get as good a control as
possible. I find it difficult to get excellent control of blood
sugars on a 24-hour basis in severe juvenile diabetics and I would
rather not have hypoglycemic episodes. Therefore, I would rather
err on the side of hyperglycemia and a little glycosuria, which I
can compensate for. It is not that I don't want to have blood
sugars of 75 to 110. In fact, I would like to have them, but you
can see what happens; it is difficult to get them unless you are

willing to risk several reactions a day. Some people even contend
that certain individuals who have experienced at least one reaction
a day over the years, do better with respect to complications than
those people who do not get these reactions. I know that's the way
Lukens feels about it. Maybe we really need a prospective study on
it. If I cannot treat someone by diet alone and the blood sugars
are such as to cause glycosuria and symptoms, I would like to use
something else. In a few instances, the sulfonylureas, or the sulfonylureas plus DBI will help me out. In other instances I definitely
need insulin because, otherwise, I will get ketoacidosis and that I
do not want to have.

DR. WOLF: I do not think anyone would disagree with you about
ketoacidosis.

DR. SPRITZ: How about the obese patient – will you permit him
to have ketosis before you use insulin?

DR. LEVINE: I would take the obese patients into a unit and
start them losing weight and then they will have controlled ketosis
under my observation for a time.

DR. SPRITZ: In other words, ketonemia is not an indication for
insulin.

DR. LEVINE: No, ketonemia per se is not.

DR. CAHILL: The hyperglycemia with the ketonemia plus the
volume collapse may be another thing.

DR. LEVINE: Yes.

DR. KNOWLES: You do not have ketosis with the negative nitrogen balance?

DR. CAHILL: No. The only concern I have with ketosis -- and
this is an aside -- is that you get a mild acidosis. That happens
on any long-range ketogenic regimen, and I am worried about calcium
stores more than nitrogen because these patients may be the osteo-
porotic-prone. Caucasian females. Therefore, I would worry that
a year or two on a ketotic diet might enhance the osteoporosis.

DR. WOLF: Have you seen anything like this in relation to the
Atkins' diet?

DR. CAHILL: We know that in the Atkins' diet there is a daily
negative calcium balance and this is something I disapprove of,
just like with long-range steroids. The results are very similar.

DR. WILLIAMS: I would like to propose what one might do if he were to decide that he did not want to use sulfonylureas or phenformin. How much of the diabetic picture, let us say, would one require before he would institute insulin treatment. To be more specific, we have already said that it is hard to know how much microangiopathy, if any, can be prevented if insulin controls hyperglycemia. So, to facilitate the discussion and to get it down to a more specific problem, although one has to consider all the facts in the case, I am wondering what this group would think of the following: if after appropriate trial of diet and exercise, you obtain fasting plasma glucose levels about 120, is it not worthwhile to then institute insulin treatment? The studies of Porte and colleagues found that you did not have your first phase of insulin release when the blood sugar was above 120 (117). In other words, this becomes a case of frank insulin deficiency. I would like to toss that out as a basis for discussion. None of us can be dogmatic but we have to make some decision.

DR. WOLF: Let me put in one question at this point, would it be important to you to measure insulin levels and glucagon in patients in order to manage them with respect to decisions of this sort?

DR. WILLIAMS: I would say that doctors throughout the world, at least so far, have not routinely been measuring those elements, but obviously the lower the level of insulin, the more will we be convinced of the need for the administration of insulin.

DR. LEVINE: Well, how sure am I if confronted by a patient with only a report on his blood sugars; how can I decide that he is insulin deficient unless I do these tests? That is, unless I check insulin levels and if you just have a dictum for the general practicing population it would not be very practical to do that. I have seen diabetics, obese diabetics, whose insulin levels were very high with blood sugars of 120 and above. So I do not have to give an obese person more insulin and I do not see any reason why I should and, if they are not obese then they will show other phenomena like proneness to ketoacidosis and so on. Therefore, I don't see how you can use a blood sugar as low as that as a criterion for the need for insulin injections.

DR. WILLIAMS: To simplify the problem let us pull out the obese factor for the moment.

Therapeutic
Preferences

DR. CAHILL: I think this will deal with the question more simply. Table 4 shows patients who are all of normal weight, divided into two groups.

TABLE 4 - Characteristics of hypothetical patients
with diabetes of varying severity and at differing
stages of life

AGE	WEIGHT	FASTING GLUCOSE	TWO HOUR GLUCOSE
GROUP A			
20	N	120	250
40	N	120	250
60	N	120	250
80	N	120	250
GROUP B			
20	N	140	300
40	N	140	300
60	N	140	300
80	N	140	300

Group A have fasting blood sugars within normal
limits. Their two hour post-prandial sugars are
in the range of 250 mg. They are ages 20, 40, 60 and 80.

Group B have fasting blood sugars of 140. Their two
hour post-prandial sugars are in the range of 300.
They have the same age distribution.

How would you treat these individuals?

DR. KNOWLES: First, I would try to get them eating properly.
I would do nothing with the patients in Group A except to educate
them on the subject of diabetes, tell them to check their urine
from time to time and examine them periodically. In Group B, even
at the age of 20 the patient is probably going to have symptoms and
I would probably start him on 20 units of Lente insulin a day. I
would do the same for the 40 year old. For those between the ages
of 60 and 80, I might use sulfonylurea "plus or minus" depending on
the results of more extensive studies. I would also consider insulin here but it may be impractical in the elderly.

DR. WILLIAMS: I would give insulin to all the patients in Group B except the 80 year old.

DR. LEVINE: I would associate myself with Dr. Knowles except that I might not even bother with sulfonylureas in the 80 year old.

DR. SPRITZ: I would not treat Group A as a group.

DR. CAHILL: We would give insulin to most of the patients in both groups except for the 80 year olds whom we would probably treat with sulfonylureas for the reasons mentioned above.

DR. LEVINE: George, what is the reason for giving insulin in the 20 and 40 year old in Group A?

DR. CAHILL: The matter of pushing harder towards trying to get and maintain a normal glycemia postprandially - just enthusiasm.

DR. LEVINE: And this would be done in expectation of doing something about the vascular problems?

DR. CAHILL: Correct, correct.

DR. LEVINE: No hard proof?

DR. CAHILL: No hard proof! No, this is a religiosity. In-deed, as far as the 20 year old is concerned, I am pretty certain that most of the people at Joslin would start him on insulin.

DR. KNOWLES: There are other reasons besides just his sugar, for starting an individual like that on treatment. This individual has to get tuned in psychologically to the fact that he has a dis-ease.

DR. WILLIAMS: Pursuing this a little further, I would like to find out what the sulfonylurea is accomplishing. In other words, is it lowering the blood sugar? Moreover, even if it does lower the blood sugar, we cannot be sure of attaining net advantages.

DR. LEVINE: What do you have to go on in addition to the blood values?

DR. WILLIAMS: I am just suggesting that we acknowledge that we do not know for sure what we are not doing. We do know that the basal insulin level before treatment with a sulfonylurea is higher than a few weeks after starting it. Therefore, you have less cir-culating insulin at least a good many hours of the day, so we have to try to decide whether the net situation adds up to a benefit or damage. This concern is over and above what side-effects may turn up as stated by the studies of the University Group (UGDP) (138).

DR. LEVINE: Bob, do you care whether the absolute level of insulin varies in one situation if the effectiveness of the insulin
is just as good or better? In other words, is the level of the hormone such a holy thing?

DR. WILLIAMS: The answer to that is the answer to the question
that I have already asked, namely, "What is the net result of giving
sulfonylurea?" The blood sugar is lowered but what is the net effect
of lowering the blood sugar on the total body metabolism?

DR. WOLF: What does the sulfonylurea do to glucagon?

DR. LEVINE: According to Samols it inhibits glucagon secretion
(123).

DR. CAHILL: Yes, in ducks.

DR. LEVINE: Also in mammals.

DR. SPRITZ: I would like to ask a critical question. Can we
do anything to preserve the vascular system of that 20 year old in
Group A. We do not have any really good reason or basis to treat
him or not to treat him. Conn's data indicates that sulfonylureas
are not helpful in restoring beta cell function (37).

DR. LEVINE: First it was said that sulfonylurea would increase
the proliferation of the beta cells but that suggestion died down.

DR. KNOWLES: Part of the UGDP study concerns a yearly glucose
tolerance test done in all patients. I think the results of the
first year have been published already showing that the blood sugars
and the weights came down (49). The sum glucose tolerance values
are being studied. It does not make any difference whether they
were on or off the drug, but in the third year the values all went
up again.

DR. CAHILL: But there was still a 15 mg% difference between
the sulfonylurea mean glucose levels and the placebo group so there
is no question that the sulfonylureas were still working.

DR. KNOWLES: Oh yes, they are still working. But that again
just reflected the enthusiasm of "doctor-and-patient" when a new
disease shows up and everybody plays ball. Then after a couple of
years the novelty wears off. The question remains why do these
three things come down and then zoom up again? And if you had to
make a guess I would put it on the basis of nutrition and perhaps
better eating habits that were practiced during those first two
years.

DR. SPRITZ: I would like to ask Harvey another question here.
Why did the 40 year old in Group B receive insulin and the 60 year
old sulfonylurea? Is that because there is something different
about the pathophysiology in that 40 year old group? Were you
worried that sulfonylurea would give him vascular disease? Or did
you base your decision on a special characteristic of his diabetes?

DR. KNOWLES: No. He was still insulin deficient. You could
start off with the sulfonylureas but their effect does not seem to
last very long at this age level and eventually they so often come
to insulin anyway. It is unusual in our Clinic to have an elderly
patient on one type of medication for more than a few years.

DR. WOLF: I would like to ask George a question here. Roger
Unger emphasized the responsiveness of
Obesity and   the alpha and beta cells to changes in
Insulin Resistance   glucose concentration and he implied
that a blunting of this responsiveness
was probably important in the process of diabetes; I think that it
is generally agreed that obese people with diabetes have a blunted
responsiveness. These same individuals when they are successfully
reduced seem to lose the blunting, or their responsiveness seems
to become better.

DR. CAHILL: Well, their insulins become lower, but whether
they regain again a first phase of release is very controversial.
There are very little hard data to show that they recapture the
same quick, brisk release as a normal person.

DR. WOLF: And is this true of the turn-off of glucagon also?

DR. CAHILL: I cannot speak to that.

DR. SPRITZ: Roger said that he did not know -- I asked him
that.

DR. LEVINE: Nobody seems to know about that.

DR. WILLIAMS: Well, they seem to lose that so-called insulin
resistance.

DR. LEVINE: Yes, but the question of the brisk, first phase
has not really been answered.

DR. CAHILL: The impression is that it does not change.

DR. WOLF: The reason that I brought this up was that I got

the impression that he did suggest that the turn-off of glucagon
was brisker in the obese diabetic patient who has lost weight. But
in any case, does this finding provide a "lead" as to how one can
begin to approach the problem of the responsiveness of the beta
cell and the alpha cell? What can you tell us about that?

DR. CAHILL: Rachmiel sees it differently from the way I look
at it. I look at it that somehow there is a global insulin resistance that is a result of increased lipid storage, and I have no
idea how the muscle knows how fat is fat, but it does know, because
it takes twice as much insulin, for example, to augment amino acid
uptake or to depress amino acid release. If you look at anything
else that insulin does, particularly with the capacity to shut off
glucose output by the liver as Phil Felig has recently explored, it
takes much more insulin to do this in the obese person (41).
So, if you make him lose weight and things come back into proportion again then all of his insulin sensitive sites throughout the
body will gain more sensitivity. That's all I know. I have no
idea what the signal for this is and I know of very little data
to suggest that the beta cell alters its pattern of response --
it just puts out less. Now the real question is, does the beta
cell undergo a kind of disuse atrophy in a normal individual as it
comes back down to normal. It's just my feeling that it does, and
I base that on Ogilvie's old observation that obese people at the
time of death have true pancreatic hyperplasia. So, if you take
any of these patients and fatten them up by using Sim's technique,
my guess is that they will have increased beta cells to match the
resistance that all this adiposity is going to create. This is
contrary to Rachmiel's concept!

DR. LEVINE: I have got to get up and point out that mysticism
is not going to do it!! The mystique is some unknown signal which
tells the pancreas that "my tissues have become resistant to insulin and therefore, you go and become hypertrophic." "And give
me some more insulin." This is the mystique that has grown up in
the literature and I cannot see this and that is the reason why
Mahler and I did some of our experiments. We first gave rats and
dogs growth hormone. This produces a hyperplasia of the islets of
Langerhans and secondly enormously increases the output of insulin.
One can observe this fact. And the third point is that insulin
resistance develops in these animals. Now, if you take these
animals and incidentally they are not obese animals, and treat
them with growth hormone for about a week to ten days with the
described results. Then if you alloxanize or give streptozotocin,
or do a pancreatectomy, and continue the administration of the
growth hormone, you will find that the insulin out-put goes down,
the hyperplasia goes down, and the insulin resistance disappears.
As a matter of fact, the insulin resistance disappears very quickly.
And then, because of these experiences, we took the ob-ob animal

which is one having genetic diabetes consisting of a hyperglycemia,
obesity and a hyperplasia with increased insulin output and insulin
resistance, but of course, this is an obese genetic animal -- and
in such an animal the administration of streptozotocin produces an
immediate responsiveness and sensitivity to insulin within two or
three days before any change in weight occurs! We postulate that
first there is a stimulus to the beta cell by either obesity or
growth hormone (or whatever). The obesity is probably due to the
food intake and whenever you have a very high insulin output you
are also putting out something which interferes with the action of
insulin in the liver or in the peripheral tissues (81).

DR. CAHILL: Rachmiel, how do you explain that the juvenile
diabetic who is hypophysectomized and requires 10 or 15 units of
insulin a day, will require 40 units of insulin a day when you give
him growth hormone.

DR. LEVINE: The explanation must be that he gets a hyperplasia
of his islets.

DR. CAHILL: The juvenile diabetic, the late twenty-year juvenile without a beta cell in his pancreas?

DR. LEVINE: I don't doubt it, and I don't know whether there
is a beta cell detectable or not. You are assuming that. It simply
appears that the islets are unable to produce some substance.

DR. SPRITZ: Ah, well, that is a mystical substance.

DR. LEVINE: The substance may be mystical but at least the
signal is there. What mystifies me about the other approach is that
you get resistance mysteriously in the periphery and that that resistance is translated into an unknown signal to produce hyperplasia
of the islets of Langerhans.

DR. SPRITZ: You are saying that the primary event is the hyperinsulinemia.

DR. CAHILL: Or "hyper-x".

DR. LEVINE: "Hyper-x" that's paralleled by insulin!

DR. SPRITZ: And O.K. "Hyper-x" in the mouse is hyperphagia -
is that right? Is that the way it works in the "ob-ob"?

DR. LEVINE: No, in the "ob-ob" it is not just hyperphagia,
because a hypothalamic mouse which has hyperphagia, has islets that
are not as hyperplastic nor as resistant as is the ob-ob animal.
I have the feeling that the difficulty in the ob-ob mouse is that

there is an absolute increase in exquisite sensitivity to the food
signal to produce hyperplasia of the pancreas. In other words, if
I were asked what the pathogenic mechanism is in the ob-ob mouse to
begin with, I would have to say that it is somewhere in the hypo-
thalamus which produces a kind of islet. Your islet and my islet is
sensitive to food, and food increases both islet number and islet
cell's size, and as George says, in an obese person you expect a
hyperplasia; Ogilvie demonstrated that years ago (93). But I
would maintain that the ob-ob animal behaves as if this same food
signal which in the ordinary person would lead to making two beta
cells, in the human it makes five or six. So in the ob-ob animal
they already start with hyperinsulinemia before there is any significant obesity.

DR. CAHILL: Rachmiel, are you suggesting, therefore, that the
insulin itself is causing the tachyphylaxis?

DR. LEVINE: It may be the insulin itself or it may be an accom-
panying material, I don't know which is which. We have tried in one
of our young animal laboratories the technique of putting insulin in
crystals in a little chamber and putting it into the mouse and produced a very high insulin level, and so far, with that very high
insulin level we have not been able to produce tachyphylaxis.

Insulin producing
Pancreatic tumors

DR. SPRITZ: Do you see this in insulinoma?

DR. CAHILL: No.

DR. LEVINE: Yes, to a certain extent you do see this. A paper
by Goldner on several insulinomas that have been observed over many
years, discusses the curious business of a poor relationship between
the insulin level and the resulting glucose level (23).

DR. CAHILL: That could have been pro-insulin.

DR. LEVINE: Yes, that could have been, but I don't know.

DR. CAHILL: But in patients having mainly insulin-producing
adenomata, you do not lose insulin sensitivity, but on the other
hand, they need so little extra insulin through an overnight fast,
just 1, or 2, or 3 micro-units per mil. to make hypoglycemia so
that you really never have a real degree of hyperinsulinemia as the
fat person does.

DR. SPRITZ: Dr. Levine, doesn't what you say fit in nicely
with Gavin's idea that increased insulin is a cause of decreased
insulin receptors (45)?

DR. LEVINE: Yes it does, but I still don't see the proof that
a receptor attachment and the biological activity are necessarily
connected. It would come out the same way. As a matter of fact,
Ron Kahn in Jesse Roth's department at the N.I.H. uses "Marder's-
Model K" tissue in his animal. But the thing that I wanted to clar-
ify just for the record, is the implication that seems to be around
in this conference and in other conferences, in relation to hormones.
Let us take those two hormones in which we are mainly interested;
the implication is that the hormones are the potent directors of the
metabolic turnovers and the metabolic direction. I would like to
correct it and I think that George Cahill would probably agree with
me that I don't know if they act this way. I want to point out that
years and years ago studies were made in a "Houssay animal", which
is a depancreatized, hypophysectomized animal. It is a very interesting experimental animal because this animal when fasted can have
a blood sugar of zero, or almost at that point, because it is incapable of mobilizing protein to make sugar during fasting. It does
not go into ketosis and help itself this way because it is incapable
of mobilizing, etc. This animal when fed is as fully diabetic as
you want to make him, that is, you give him a lot of protein and
his liver has no problems in making sugar and making urea. Years
ago I gave them fatty acids directly, or at least some form of fatty
acids directly, and one can get ketones. Nowadays one should re-do
this quantitatively. The point that I am trying to make is that
this animal has no insulin and, as far as I know, he has no glucagon
unless the gut makes one or both of these hormones.

In such an animal without any of the hormones, when he is given
protein (which means that he gets amino acids because that is the
way it is absorbed) he finds no difficulty with gluconeogenesis at
all, without having these hormones. And, therefore, the substrate
directly affects the function of the liver. We sometimes place too
much stress on the hormones as being responsible for, and directing,
the whole situation. I can see that George is smiling.

DR. CAHILL: I have to agree because we have one animal that
does it. He does exactly this; he eats his own weight in pure protein within 30 minutes. This is the vampire bat. Then he has to
discharge all of the urea in water before he can fly again, and
that bat has a tremendous catabolic rate and we can find no change
in either insulin or glucagon levels. It is all a function of
amino acid concentration that is absorbed into its gut. So it is
always poised to handle protein catabolically and does not change.
And that is why I was smiling when you were discussing this matter.

DR. LEVINE: In other words, how much are we over-emphasizing
the roles of the endocrines?

DR. WOLF: This leads us very naturally to another topic that

we should get on the record. That is that before we had insulin,
                              the management of diabetes was exclusively
Dietary Therapy   by diet. Since the advent of insulin
                              therapy, the prevailing preferences in
dietary management have differed from time to time. Could we say a
few words about the rationale of dietary selection? What do you do,
Harvey?

DR. KNOWLES: It depends on which clinic I happen to be in. Are
you asking me this question in the treatment of diabetes in general?

DR. WOLF: Yes, where are your landmarks?

DR. KNOWLES: Well, I do what is customary in this country, "not
knowing what I'm doing." First, let us come to the calories. The
landmark in calories is to reduce the overweight person and if, on
the other hand, they are undernourished, to bring them up to optimum
weight. I don't know what that is, but I use the desirable weight
tables and adjust to age, body frame and sex. That is number one.
Number two is to count the 24-hour composition of the intake. We
use something that approaches the A.D.A. exchange system. Actually
it is the 40-20-40 ratio per total 24-hour composition. I must say
here that I do that because that is what seems to be the diet cus-
tom in the United States today. And I don't know whether what we
eat in the United States today is what we were destined to eat. Of
course if we were going back 100,000 years to the advent of agricul-
ture, supposed to be 10 thousand years B.C., as Dr. Margaret Albrink
said, in those days you killed an animal once a month and then star-
ved until the next month and killed another animal ... or the animal
killed you! (2)

DR. SPRITZ: I thought he said that was before the Roosevelt
administration!!

DR. KNOWLES: But this is what we use merely because it is what
is used in America today. I have mentioned calories and I have mentioned 24-hour composition of the total intake of food. Thirdly,
we spread it out so that there will be three major periods of food
consumption per day plus a snack at bedtime in all except the elderly
and some long-standing juvenile diabetics (who do not seem to need
them) and in younger persons who probably have to have a mid-afternoon snack. But there is regularity, particularly for the insulin-
dependent patient because he has to eat in order to match his insulin level -- there are no ifs or buts about it. So generally
this is what is done -- I believe this is what is done in all diabetic clinics.

But I must backtrack and say that I do not know what optimum
weight should be for optimum life activity; secondly, I do not know
what should be the optimum ratio of the three foodstuffs we eat —

carbohydrates, proteins and fats -- in order to give us the maximum
output of productivity and longevity.

DR. WILLIAMS: What do you do in general about the ratio of
carbohydrate and fat?

DR. KNOWLES: Do you mean that the proportion of calories sup-
plied by fat in the diet should be 40% or 35% or lower?

DR. WILLIAMS: We generally use 40% or something close to it.

DR. KNOWLES: We have not changed it in the environment that I
am in. In the first place as I discussed yesterday, the juvenile
diabetics we have are on an unmeasured diet system. It is an entirely different phenomenon. In fact, they have more dietary interviews,
more dietary instruction than given in our regular diabetic clinic.
The patients just do not measure, but I am constantly looking at
their intake. What the American adult patient is eating today is
extremely difficult to determine, let alone the teenager. We have
stayed with the 40-20-40 ratio in our population which is, however,
indigent. If I get down to a 35% fat, the diets just do not appeal
to the kids. At 30% fat, we could not get our clinic population to
really go along with it; they just do not like it. Of course this
is the lower income class patient and lower education level group.
Perhaps in the upper levels that George Cahill or Norty Spritz sees,
you can do better.

DR. WILLIAMS: But you do attempt to eliminate free sugar such
as candy bars, coca-colas and so forth?

DR. KNOWLES: No, not if they are grossly part of the intake.
I have not restricted sucrose, nor done anything really. If we can
get our diabetic patients to eat three meals a day at the right
time, we feel we are doing pretty well. Of course, we do not preach
this but this is what happens.

DR. WILLIAMS: We encourage patients who are on Lente or NPH
insulin to eat mid-morning, mid-afternoon and at bedtime, because
the rate of insulin absorption has no relationship to whether or
not you are taking food. And I know, at least, that it protects
against hypoglycemic reactions. Whether the net result is good or
bad, it is hard to say.

DR. WOLF: In talking about evidence and rational basis for the
dietary manipulation, Harvey has mentioned acceptability and Bob
has mentioned covering insulin. What other firm evidence do we have?
For example, you suggested the prohibition of candy bars. What can
you tell us about that? In other words, why is that a good thing?

DR. WILLIAMS: In those patients who spill sugar, eating candy-bars would cause them to spill more. But of course the result is a change of equilibrium over a short time. We do not know whether or not it tends to cause damage.

DR. CAHILL: Is it reasonable to give insulin to lower glucose and then allow the intake of foods which can drive glucose up to tremendous levels very rapidly in some of these cases, especially when they are a little low in insulin? I am talking about not restricting carbohydrates (candy bars) and I am being very blunt here. In other words, you want to maintain favor with the kids, realizing they are probably going to do it anyway. In short, I am asking if this is not a kind of hypocrisy; probably with a good purpose in mind, but nevertheless a physiological hypocrisy?

DR. KNOWLES: You may have something.

DR. CAHILL: Yes, but you see what I am driving at.

DR. WOLF: Yesterday, we heard about the great variation in the giving of glucose along with the long-lasting insulins.

DR. KNOWLES: This program and the one that Dr. Cahill refers to is the one that I still regard as an experimental program that was started in 1932, before I got into the picture in the mid-40s. As the years went by, I did not see any need to change it and I cannot do that until you show me that another program will give a better result. When anybody does that, I will be the first one to move over to it. Every patient who goes into this program still goes in as an experimental subject since I am a minority in the country in what I am doing by far. They all get the "pros and cons". Every child (6 to 8) starts at the Children's Hospital and then when they reach the age of 16 they come over to me for the long term treatment.

DR. CAHILL: Well before you start, do you believe that hyperglycemia is bad?

DR. KNOWLES: I do not know, and I have no beliefs at all.

DR. CAHILL: You say that would require a very rigid approach and you say, "I cannot accept" but you can still have a visceral feeling on the issue without having the facts to back it up.

DR. KNOWLES: Yes, I agree. I feel that it is bad.

DR. CAHILL: How about the microvascular disease?

DR. KNOWLES: It is not a matter of belief, it is that I just don't know, George.

DR. WILLIAMS: Would not Spiro's studies suggest that allowing marked hyperglycemia is manufacturing more vascular disease? (129)

DR. KNOWLES: Yes, there are a hundred things that "suggest" it.

DR. LEVINE: Then you must ask, "Why is not his incidence of retinopathy different from any other program study?"

DR. WILLIAMS: It may be.

DR. LEVINE: It is not.

DR. WILLIAMS: We do not know and it is hard to quantitate that.

DR. KNOWLES: I do not have anybody to match data with because I have never been able to get any other Center to do prospective data studies like ours. The one that I have mentioned, Hirohata, deals with mortality only. (57).

DR. LEVINE: Yes, but their findings coincided with yours.

DR. KNOWLES: Those are the only two that I know of.

DR. WILLIAMS: Why do you add item 4 in the light of the statements you made?

DR. KNOWLES: I said, "Excess."

DR. WILLIAMS: Is a candy bar excess?

DR. KNOWLES: No, because that may be part of the afternoon snack and as long as it is a coca-cola every day at 4:00 p.m., or when they come home from school. These teenagers, with their sports in school, playing football, and so on, have to eat before supper because they cannot hold out. It may be a coke and cheese and crackers, and at bedtime it may be a coke, just as long as they stick to a uniform regimen one can control them.

DR. WILLIAMS: Would you not also try to get in some more protein in these kids because they are wasting protein — they are burning it up — they have gluconeogenesis.

DR. LEVINE: A diabetic, even an insulin-deficient diabetic, who is being treated with diet and insulin has little, if any, wastage of protein compared with the non-diabetic.

DR. WILLIAMS: Where then does he get his high blood sugar from midnight to around breakfast-time?

DR. LEVINE: Oh, they have stores in the form of glycogen and they do not become gluconeogenetic just over-night. As a matter of fact also, the urea excretion is not any different from normals, but of course if they have not been treated that is a different story.

DR. WILLIAMS: But quite often you do not get enough insulin in there to cause complete utilization.

DR. LEVINE: I have never seen any evidence that there is not enough insulin to maintain a normal nitrogen balance.

DR. KNOWLES: You remember the old studies of Dunlop when he purposely made them symptomatic (as polyuric and hyperglycemic) and then he measured his glucose intake and output (44). And the utilization rates were shown to be normal. The problem, though, was whether the pathway was physiologic. I have two dietitians, one of them at the Children's Hospital and the other at the Cincinnati General, and every time they come in we go over this thing with all sorts of discussion. Regardless of the amount of education, I think we do more to get normal eating habits than are done in the average diabetic clinic in this country.

DR. CAHILL: Yes, but Harvey what you are presenting here is that while it is true that you are giving liberal carbohydrates, you are really trying to get precise daily patterns -- a very good goal.

DR. KNOWLES: Yes, this is very good, but you see I am always called the "free dieter" in this country, and there is really no such thing. They just don't measure their intake. But the juvenile diabetic has to follow a pattern.

DR. CAHILL: Yes, but it is really a very carefully restricted pattern.

DR. KNOWLES: Yes, but without the stigma of diabetes. We did this aiming towards normal nutrition. You just serve up a tray to a patient with a diabetic sign, and he will not eat it. If you give this to him without the sign and tell him to eat it, then perhaps you will get cooperation.

DR. WILLIAMS: There is one additional point I wanted to comment on. Three of the five types of Frederickson's hyperlipidemias are associated with an increased incidence of diabetes. Some of these have various enzymatic genetic deficiencies, etc. For this reason we keep a check on the triglyceride and cholesterol levels, more especially the triglycerides. In such instances, after good insulin treatment, if we find that the triglycerides remain up, we often lower their fats and increase their carbohydrates.

DR. WOLF: What you are saying is that you are treating hyperlipidemia.

DR. WILLIAMS: Yes.

DR. SPRITZ: Is that the way to treat it?

DR. WILLIAMS: The hyperlipidemia is due in large part to the
carbohydrates because then the liver puts out more lipids. But,
let me say this, with the markedly untreated case of juvenile diabetes, you always have lipoprotein lipase deficiency. Then when
you treat them with insulin, in a great many you will get that back
up to normal. However, some of them have a genetic abnormality of
lipoprotein lipase and in those cases insulin does not correct it.
Therefore, one has to deal with a problem like that from a dietary
viewpoint by restricting the intake of fat.

DR. KNOWLES: Of course that is one of the theoretical reasons
for control of the diet. There are hundreds of things you can do.
As a matter of fact, this study took about five years in order to
get across that home interviews with the parents of the patients
were needed. As I told you before, I had a nurse who spent a lot
of time with them, and a dietitian whose purpose was to go around
visiting and talking with aunts, uncles and anybody else she could
contact. Actually, when we came down to the mean composition of the
intake, the proportions of protein, carbohydrate and fat that we
found to be in the average American diet - the average protein was
in the neighborhood of 17%.

DR. SPRITZ: Those are in caloric proportions.

DR. KNOWLES: We found that the patients were eating just about
average American meals.

DR. SPRITZ: It is very hard to get Americans to deviate from
that pattern. I think that yours is not the only experience with
that. There have been a lot of attempts and instruction to try to
get them away from that pattern, and when you analyze what they
eat, it is very different.

DR. LEVINE: You know it is very difficult. I consider it as
one of the great accomplishments of my years at Michael Reese Hospital in Chicago, where the diet menu had 400 pages that I reduced
it to 32 pages. Because all of this maneuvering is within a very
narrow range. You need a certain amount of protein and I do not
care whether you are diabetic or not. This is about 3/4 to 1 gram
per kilo, and then all you can do is to maneuver the carbohydrates

and fat and you cannot go below a certain amount of fat because it
is dry stuff that nobody will eat.

DR. SPRITZ: I am not even sure that you should.

DR. LEVINE: Whether you should or not, you really cannot do
it as patients will not tolerate it.

DR. SPRITZ: I think Bob has made the point that diet manipulation in the diabetic patient does not
have much to do with the diabetes directly. When you treat obesity, you
treat it as best you can with dietary
manipulation. And you treat hyperlipidemia of the various sorts
with dietary manipulation, which is very difficult. And Bob is
talking about decreasing fat in some hypertriglyceridemics. Sometimes that works but more often decreasing carbohydrate in these
patients will decrease their plasma lipid levels.

The treatment of
Hyperlipidemia

DR. CAHILL: How about polyunsaturated fats? I would like to
hear Dr. Spritz's opinion.

DR. SPRITZ: As a general principle, we see the presence of
diabetes as an added risk factor. The general strategy of dealing
with these added risk factors is that the more there are, the more
vigorously you deal with as many as you can. For instance, the diabetic patient who smokes has a double disadvantage in his risk of
developing coronary artery disease. Similarly a diabetic patient
with hyperbetalipoproteinemia has an exaggerated risk of atherosclerosis. A diabetic patient with an elevated triglyceride concentration, in most instances, should lose weight. But in some patients
mild carbohydrate restriction, and in some other patients, ethanol
restriction, are the keys to the hypertriglyceridemia, and I am very
quick to treat them with drugs if diet does not succeed in altering
their plasma lipids.

DR. LEVINE: You are referring now, I guess, to atromid.

DR. SPRITZ: For the hypertriglyceridemic patients, atromid is
probably the first line drug. And for the hypercholesterolemia
patients, the resins such as cholestyramine and so forth.

DR. CAHILL: How about nicotinic acid?

DR. SPRITZ: In young people with Type 2 hypercholesterolemia,
it might help. But we have had bad experiences because we do not
get very good patient compliance with nicotinic acid in adult patient
with Type 2 disease. I think they do better with cholestyramine and
atromid together. But you know, everybody does it differently. It

is a very lithogenic combination, by the way.

DR. KNOWLES: We started about ten years ago or more, sometime around 1960, with that sort of approach and look upon it as a sort of wishful thinking.

DR. WOLF: Explain that to us.

DR. KNOWLES: Well, we are emphasizing to patients more poultry and cutting down on red meat which is easy nowadays because the people I deal with just cannot afford it anyway. The emphasis on the high polyunsaturated cooking oils, margarine and then the weight problem that Dr. Spritz mentioned, are not problems in juvenile diabetics because it is unusual to have, so I do not have to go overboard on that as much as you who are dealing with adults. I have about 400 juveniles and we are a lipoprotein screening center. I wonder what your experience is, George. Has anyone done a study on the patterns of lipoproteins seen in these Centers of large juvenile diabetic groups.

DR. CAHILL: They are usually discouragingly normal. I should say, nicely normal, but we are looking for abnormal patterns.

DR. KNOWLES: I have two or three with Type 2, but the families have Type 2 also. So maybe it is a genetic pattern.

DR. LEVINE: No, it is in the adult diabetic, the prebetalipoprotein.

DR. SPRITZ: That is right, Type 2 is in the adult.

DR. CAHILL: In fact, even the juvenile type of diabetic who has had 20 to 25 years of the disease with his coronary and triopathy (eye, kidney and nerve) still seems to have normal lipids. So this makes it highly difficult to indict the lipids except in the older diabetic.

DR. LEVINE: There has been a tendency in the last 15–20 years particularly in the last 10 years, to make the diagnosis of diabetes more and more permissive. In making the criteria less rigid, more and more people become classified as diabetics and so the prevalence figures go up. I am wondering whether it is time to go the other way round and make the criteria more rigid and define this disorder by something that is more palpable than a statement such as, "If in the second hour of a glucose tolerance test the blood sugar is 141, then this is diabetes." How do you feel about that, George?

DR. CAHILL: Yes it is like how tall is tall? Is it 6'1" or 6'2" or 5'11"? It is purely empirical.

DR. SPRITZ: Even more important is the fact that if we have nothing to offer these people whom we classify as diabetics, at least we should be reluctant to do so.

DR. WOLF: That is why I raised the issue, namely, what is the benefit of early detection? What are the dividends to the patient? Apparently we have little to offer the recently discovered "chemical" diabetic except to arouse his anxiety and perhaps to expose him to promiscuous therapeutic measures.

SUMMARY

DR. WOLF: The discussions of the last two and a half days
have described what is really an explosion of new data with respect
to diabetes. Nevertheless, until an effective synthesis of the new
findings can be achieved, the management of patients with diabetes
remains at an empirical level. The complex metabolic interactions
that characterize diabetes are being sorted out but their relationship to the appearance of structural vascular lesions remains obs-
cure. The problem of reconciling the morphologic, chemical, epidemiological and clinical evidence into a cohesive whole may be dealt
with more effectively in the future as studies of the ultrastructure
of islet cells in healthy humans are supplemented by data from the
juvenile-onset and the adult diabetic.

Very important evidence was presented of regulatory inter-
connections of the alpha and beta cells of the islets by way of
gap junctions between adjacent cells in the pancreas. Moreover
there are indications that under certain circumstances remodeling
of intercellular membrane junctions occurs so that a gap junction
may be replaced by a tight junction. It appears that these islet
structures may be disturbed in a variety of ways. Recent data
support earlier etiologic hints that a genetic proclivity may be
triggered by a viral infection and perhaps by other stresses as
well. Potentially pathogenic mechanisms may include altered end-
organ responsiveness to insulin and glucagon as well as defective
signals for the elaboration of these hormones and defective signal-
ing equipment for turn-on and turn-off of insulin and glucagon.
Suggestive evidence is emerging that the endothelial cells of the
capillaries may participate in the signalling process.

It was not emphasized in the discussion but was frequently
referred to, that many of the regulatory processes are fundamentally
subject to control by the central nervous system. The endocrine
organs including adrenal gland may serve to mediate some of the
effects. Those mediated by the autonomic nerves would be less
readily detected. One can measure the concentration of circulating
regulatory hormones but evidence of effects of local neurotransmitters is difficult to adduce because the neurotransmitters are
promptly eliminated in situ and do not gain access to the blood
in significant quantity. Thus measurements of blood concentration
of norepinephrine, for example, or other substances are not trans-
latable into the amount of sympathetic nerve activity in the vis-
cera or blood vessels.

Of what significance are the illuminating discussions in this
Colloquium to the practicing physician?

First of all, he is warned that glucose intolerance (chemical

diabetes) is not necessarily a progressive disorder, especially in
the elderly, and requires no therapy other than reduction to "ideal"
weight. The hazards of overdosing with insulin are emphasized,
especially the potentially damaging effects of hypoglycemia to the
brain and the catabolic consequences of insulin provoked glucagonemia.

Next, although not of immediate practical significance, the
practitioner is made aware of the importance of glucagon and of
the finely tuned reciprocal relationship of glucagon and insulin.
He may also look forward to rapidly unfolding new developments that
may direct future therapy toward suppressing excessive glucagon
production or toward modifying the alpha-beta cell signalling system.

Finally, as our developing understanding of the widespread
systemic disease, diabetes, was put into a historical perspective
many important lacunae in our present knowledge became identifiable. At present there is no room for dogmatic positions on etiology or therapy, but for the near future there is a bright prospect
of a far more comprehensive grasp of this important clinical condition.

BIBLIOGRAPHY

1. Alberti, K.G.M.M., Christensone, N.J., et al.: Inhibition of
    insulin secretion by somatostatin. Lancet 2: 1299, 1973.

2. Albrink, M.J.: Carbohydrate metabolism in cardiovascular dis-
    ease. Annals Int. Med. 62: 6, 1330-1333, 1965.

3. Allen, F.M.: Current judgments on metabolic control and compli-
    cations of diabetes. N. Eng. J. Med. 248: 133, 1953.

4. Andersson, A.: Effects of glucose on the structure and meta-
    bolism of isolated pancreatic islets maintained in tissue
    culture. Uppsala Dissertations from the Faculty of Med.,
    Stockholm, Sweden, 1973.

5. Bagdade, J.D., Porte, D., and Bierman, E.L.: Diabetic Lipemia.
    N. Eng. J. Med. 276: 427, 1967.

6. Becker, D., Miller, M.: Presence of diabetic glomerulosclerosis
    in patients with hemochromatosis. N. Eng. J. Med. 263:
    367, 1960.

7. Beisswenger, P.J., and Spiro, R.G.: Studies on the human glome-
    rular basement membrane. Composition, nature of the carbo-
    hydrate units and chemical changes in diabetes mellitus.
    Diabetes 22: 180, 1973.

8. Bennett, M.V.L.: Function of electrotonic junctions in embryonic
    and adult tissues. Fed. Proc. 32, 65-75, 1973.

9. Bloodworth, J.M.B.: Diabetic Retinopathy. Diabetes, 11: 1-22,
    1962.

10. Bloodworth, J.M.B., Sommers, S.C.: Cirrhotic glomerulosclerosis
    a renal lesion associated with hepatic cirrhosis. Lab.
    Invest. 8: 962-978, 1959.

11. Bouchardat, A.: De la glycosurie on Diabète Sucre. Libr.
    Germer Bailliere, Paris, 1875.

12. Braaten, J.T., Schenk, A., Lee, M.J., McGuigan, J.E., and
    Mintz, D.H.: Cyclic nucleotide-mediated secretion of
    glucagon and gastrin in monolayer culture of rat pancreas.
    J. Clin. Invest. 53: 10a, 1974.

13. Branton, D.: Fracture faces of frozen membranes. Proc. Natl.
    Acad. Sc. (Washington) 55: 1048-1056, 1966.

14. Brazeau, P., Rivier, J., et al.: Inhibition of growth hormone
       secretion in the rat by synthetic somatostatin. Endocrin.
       94: 184, 1974.

15. Bruner, J.C.: Experimenta nova crica pancreas. Amsterdam,
       1682.

16. Borchardt, L.: Die hypophysenglykosurie und ihre beziehung
       zum diabetes bei der akromegalie. Ztschr. F. Klin. Med.
       66: 332-348, 1908.

17. Burton, T.Y., Kearns, T.P., and Rynearson, E.H.: Diabetic
       retinopathy following total pancreatectomy. Mayo Clinic
       Proc., 32: 735-739, 1957.

18. Cahill, G.: Unpublished data.

19. Cawley, T.: A singular case of diabetes, consisting entirely
       in the quality of the urine, with an inquiry into the
       different theories of that disease. London Med. J.,
       9: 286-308, 1788.

20. Cerasi, E. and Luft, R.: The plasma insulin response to glu-
       cose infusion in healthy subjects and in diabetes mellitus.
       Acta Endocrin. 55: 278-304, 1967.

21. Cerasi, E., Luft, R., Efendric, S.: Decreased sensitivity of
       the pancreatic beta cells to glucose in prediabetic and
       diabetic subjects. Diabetes, 21: 224, 1972.

22. Cherrington, A., Vranic, M., Fono, P., and Kovacevic, N.:
       Effect of glucagon on glucose turnover and plasma free
       fatty acids in depancreatized dogs maintained on matched
       insulin infusions. Canadian J. Physiol. Pharmacol.,
       50: 946-954, 1972.

23. Chowdhury, F., Bleicher, J.: Studies of tumor hypoglycemia.
       Metabolism, 22: 663-674, 1973.

24. Conard, V., Legros, F.: Insulin adsorption to cell membrane
       of an autotrophic marine alga. Diabetes 23 (Supp. 1),
       368, 1974.

25. Creutzfeld, W.: in Handbook of Diabetes Mellitus, (E. F.
       Pfeiffer, ed.) Lehmanns Verlag, Munich, 239, 1971.

26. Deamer, D.W., Leonard, R., Tardieu, A., and Branton, D.:
       Lamellar and hexagonal lipid phases visualized by freeze-
       etching. Biochim et Biophys. Acta 219: 47-60, 1970.

27. DeWulf, H., and Hers, H.G.: The role of glucose, glucagon and
     glucocorticoids in the regulation of liver glycogen syn-
     thesis. European J. Biochem. 6: 558-564, 1968.

28. Dobbs, R., Sakurai, H., Sasaki, H., Faloona, G., Valverde, I.,
     Baetens, D., Orci, L., and Unger, R.: Glucagon - Role in
     the hyperglycemia of diabetes mellitus. Science, 187:
     544-547, 1975.

29. Dobson, M.: Medical Observations and Inquiries. Vol. 259,
     London, 1776.

30. Dudrick, S.J., Long, J.M., and Steiger, E.: Intravenous hyper-
     alimentation. Med. Clin. N. Amer. 84: 577, 1970.

31. Duff, G.L. and MacMillan, G.C.: The effect of alloxan diabetes
     on experimental cholesterol atherosclerosis in the rabbit.
     J. Exptl. Med. 89: 611-630, 1949.

32. Eisenstein, A.B. and Strack, I.: Effect of high protein feed-
     ing on gluconeogenesis in rat liver. Diabetes, 20: 577-
     585, 1971.

33. Engelson, G.: Studies in diabetes mellitus. Acta Ped. Vol.
     43 (Supp. 97): 1, 1954.

34. Engstrom, L.H.: Structure in the erythrocyte membrane.
     Dissertation Abstracts Int. 3871-B, 1971.

35. Evans, D.J.: Generalized islet-hypertrophy and beta cell
     hyperplasia in a case of long term juvenile diabetes.
     Diabetes, 21: 114, 1972.

36. Fajans, S.S. and Conn, J.W.: An approach to the prediction of
     diabetes mellitus by modification of the glucose tolerance
     test with cortisone. Diabetes, 3: 296-304, 1954.

37. Fajans, S.S., Floyd, J.C., Pok, S. and Conn, J.W.: The course
     of asymptomatic diabetes in young people. Tr. Assn. Am.
     Phys., 82: 211, 1969.

38. Fajans, S.S., Floyd, J.C., Taylor, C.I. and Pek, S.: Hetero-
     geneity of insulin responses in latent diabetes. Trans.
     Assn. Am. Phys., 87: 83-94, 1974.

39. Farquhar, M.G. and Palade, G.E.: Junctional complexes in
     various epithelia. J. Cell Biol. 17: 375-412, 1963.

40. Feldherr, C.M.: Advances in cell and molecular biology (E.S.
     Du Praw, ed.) Academic Press, New York and London, 273-307,
     1972.

41. Felig, P., Wahren, J., Hendler, R. and Brundin, T.: Splanchnic
     glucose and amino acid metabolism in obesity. J. Clin.
     Invest. 53: 582-590, 1974.

42. Ferner, H.: Das iselsystem des pankreas. Entwicklung, histo-
     biologie, und pathophysiologie. Mit besondgrer berucksichti-
     gung des diabetes mellitus. G. Thieme, Stuttgart, p. 119,
     1952.

43. Forssmann, W.G., Orci, L., Pictet, R., Renold, A.E. and
     Rouiller, C.: The endocrine cells in the epithelium of
     the gastrointestinal mucosa of the rat. J. Cell Biol.
     40: 692-715, 1969.

44. Forsyth, C.C., Kinnear, T.W.G., Dunlop, D.M.: Diet in Diabetes.
     Brit. Med. J., 1: 1095, 1951.

45. Gavin, J.R., Roth, J., Neville, D.M., DeMeyts, P. and Buell,
     D.N.: Insulin dependent regulation of insulin receptor
     concentrations: A direct demonstration in cell culture.
     Proc. Nat. Acad. Sci., 71: 84, 1974.

46. Gepts, W.: In Handbook of Physiology, Section 7, 289-303.
     (D. F. Steiner and N. Freinkel, eds.) Washington, D.C.,
     American Physiological Society, 1972.

47. Gepts, W.: Pathologic anatomy of the pancreas in juvenile
     diabetes mellitus. Diabetes, 14: 619, 1965.

48. Gilula, N.B., Reeves, O.R. and Steinbach, A.: Metabolic coup-
     ling, ionic coupling and cell contacts. Nature, London,
     235: 262-265, 1972.

49. Goldner, M.G., Knatterud, G.L. and Prout, T.E.: Effects of
     hypoglemic agents on vascular complications in patients
     with adult-onset diabetes. J. Am. Med. Assn. 218: 1400-
     1410, 1971.

50. Goldstein, S., Littlefield, J.W. and Soeldner, J.J.: Diabetes
     mellitus and aging: Diminished plating efficiency of cul-
     tured human fibroblasts. Proc. Natl. Acad. Sci. 64: 155,
     1969.

51. Goldstein, S., Niewiarowski, S. and Singal, D.P.: Pathological
     implications of cell aging in vitro. Fed. Proc. 34: 56-63,
     1975.

52. Goodner, C.J., Ensinck, J.W., Chideckel, E., Palmer, J.,
       Koerker, D.J., Ruch, W. and Gale, C.C.: Somatostatin,
       a hypothalamic inhibitor of the endocrine pancreas.
       J. Clin. Invest. 53: 28a, 1974.

53. Goto, Y., and Fukuhara, N.: Causes of death in 933 diabetic
       autopsy cases. J. Jap. Diabetic Soc. 11: 197, 1968.

54. Greider, M.H. and McGuigan, J.E.: A comparison of ulcerogenic
       tumors of the pancreas with the gastrin cell of normal
       human pancreas and hog antrum. Am. J. Pathol. 59: 76a-
       77a, 1970.

55. Hanse, A.P. and Johanssen, K.: Diurnal patterns of blood glu-
       cose, serum-free fatty acids, insulin, glucagon, and
       growth hormone in normals and juvenile diabetics.
       Diabetalogia 6: 27, 1969.

56. Hayflick, L.: The limited in vitro lifetime of human diploid
       cell strains. Exptl. Cell Res. 37: 614, 1965.

57. Hirohata, T., MacMahon, B., Root, H.F.: The Natural History
       of Diabetes. I. Mortality. Diabetes (16) 12: 875-881,
       1967.

58. Hirschberg, M., Deutsche Med. Wchschr. 17ff (1887). 51ff (1890)
       13 (1891).

59. Houssay, B.A.: Carbohydrate metabolism. New Eng. J. Med.,
       214: 971-986, 1936.

60. Huff, J.C., Hierholzer, J.C. and Farris, W.A.: An "outbreak"
       of juvenile diabetes mellitus: Consideration of a viral
       etiology. Am. J. Epidemiol. 100 (4): 277-287, 1974.

61. Hutchison, H.T., Werrbach, K., Vance, C. and Haber, B.: Up-
       take of neurotransmitters by clonal lines of astrocytoma
       and neuroblastoma in culture. I. Transport of γ-amino-
       butyric acid. Brain Res. 66: 265-274, 1974.

62. Johnson, D.G. and Ensinck, J.W. et al.: Inhibition of glucagon
       and insulin secretion by somatostatin in the rat pancreas
       perfused in situ. To be published.

63. Johnson, R.G. and Sheridan, J.D.: Junctions between cancer
       cells in culture. Ultrastructure and permeability.
       Science 174:717-719, 1971.

64. Johnsson, S.: Retinopathy and nephropathy in diabetes melli-
         tus: Comparison of the effects of two forms of treatment.
         Diabetes, 9: 1, 1-8, 1960.

65. Kilo, C., Vogler, N., Williamson, J.R.: Muscle capillary base-
         ment membrane changes related to aging and to diabetes
         mellitus. Diabetes, Vol 21,8: 881-905, 1972.

66. Kimball, C.P. and Murlin, J. R.: Aqueous extracts of pancreas.
         III. Some precipitation reactions of insulin. J. Biol.
         Chem. 58: 337, 1923.

67. Knopf, R.F., Fajans, S.S., Floyd, J.C., Pek, S. and Conn, J.W.:
         Elevated "casual" fasting plasma levels of growth hormone
         (GH) in patients with diabetic retinopathy (DR).
         Diabetes, 21: 322, 1972.

68. Koerker, D.J. and Ruch, W. et al. : Somatostatin: Hypothalamic
         inhibitor of the endocrine pancreas. Science, 184: 482,
         1974.

69. Kreines, K., Kim, O. and Knowles, H. C.: Glomerulosclerosis,
         hemochromatosis and diabetes mellitus. Am. J. Clin. Path.
         54: 47-52, 1970.

70. Kreutziger, G.O.: Freeze-etching of intercellular junctions
         of mouse liver. In Proc. 26th Electron Microscop. Soc.
         Amer., Claitor's Publishing Division, Baton Rouge, La.,
         234-235, 1968.

71. Kummerle, F., Beck, K. and Tenner, R.: V'vere Senza pancreas
         Minerva Med. 61: 265-269, 1970.

72. Laguesse, E. : Sur la formation des ilots de Langerhans dans
         le pancreas. Compt. Rend. Soc. Biol. 45: 819, 1893.

73. Lawrence, R.D.: Treatment of 90 severe diabetics with soluble
         insulin for 20-40 years. Effect of Diabetic Control on
         Complications. Brit. Med. J. 2: 1624, 1963.

74. LeFebrve, P.J. and Unger, R.H.(eds). In Glucagon, Pergamon
         Press, 1972.

75. Leffert, H.L,: Growth control of primary cultured fetal rat
         hepatocytes. VI. Hormonal control of DNA synthesis and
         its possible significance to the problem of liver regener-
         ation. In press.

76. Levine, R.: Symposium on Microangiopathy. Diabetes, 13:
        420, 1964.

77. Like, A.A. and Orci, L.: Embryogenesis of the human pancreatic
        islets: A light and electron microscopic study. Diabetes,
        21 (Suppl. 2) 511-534, 1972.

78. Lindner, A., Clarra, B., Shearand, D.J. and Scribner, B.H.:
        Accelerated atherosclerosis in prolonged maintenance hemo-
        dialysis. N. Eng. J. Med., 290: 697, 1974.

79. Logothetopolous, J.: In Handbook of Physiology, (D. F. Steiner
        and N. Frenkel, eds.) Volume I, 67-76, 1972.

80. Lukens, F.D.W., Dohan, F.C. and Wolcott, M.W.: Pituitary dia-
        betes in the cat: recovery following phlorhizin treatment.
        Endocrinology, 32: 475-487, 1943.

81. Mahler, R.J.: The pathogenesis of pancreatic islet cell hyper-
        plasia and insulin insensitivity in obesity. Adv. Met.
        Disorders, 7: 213-241, 1974.

82. Malaisse, W., Malaisse-Lagae, F., Gerritsen, G.C., Dulin, W.E.
        and Wright, P.H.: Insulin secretion in vitro by the
        pancreas of the Chinese hamster. Diabetologia, 3: 109-
        114, 1967.

83. Manganiello, V. and Vaughan, M.: Selective loss of adipose
        cell responsiveness to glucagon with growth in the rat.
        J. Lipid Res., 13: 12, 1972.

84. Mauer, S.M., Sutherland, E.R., Steffers, M.W., Leonard, R.J.,
        Najarian, J.J., Michael, A.F. and Brown, D.M.: Pancreatic
        islet transplantation. Effects on the glomerular lesions
        of experimental diabetes in the rat. Diabetes, 23:
        748-753, 1974.

85. McNutt, N.S. and Weinstein, R.S.: In: Progress in Biophys.
        and Molecular Biology. (J.A.V. Butler and D. Noble, eds.)
        Pergamon Press, London, Vol. 26: 45-101, 1973.

86. Meyer, H.W. and Winkelmann, H.: Uber die anordnung der membran
        proteine nach untersuchungen mit der gefrieratzung an
        isolierten erythrozytenmembranen. Protoplasma, 75: 255-
        284, 1972.

87. Mirsky, I.A.: The influence of insulin on the protein metabo-
        lism of nephrectomized dogs. Am. J. Physiol. 124: 569, 1938.

88. Moor, H. and Muhlethaler, K.J.: Fine structure in frozen-etched
     yeast cells. J. Cell Biol., 17: 609-628, 1963.

89. Najarian, J.S., Henriksen, A.I., Simmons, R.L.and Kjellstrend,
     C.M.: Kidney transplantation for patients with diabetes
     mellitus. Transplant. Proc. 6: 4, 121-126, 1974.

90. Najarian, J.S., Kjellstrend, C.M., Simmons, R.L., Buselmeier,
     T.J., von Hartitzsch, B. and Goetz, S.C.: Renal transplan-
     tation for diabetic glomerulosclerosis. Ann. Surg.,
     178:4, 477-483, 1973.

91. Naunyn, B.: Diabetes Mellitus, Holder, Vienna, 1898.

92. New, M.I., Roberts, T.N., Bierman, E.L. and Reader, G.C.:
     The significance of blood lipid alterations in diabetes
     mellitus. Diabetes 12: 208, 1963.

93. Ogilvie, R.F.: A quantitative estimation of the pancreatic
     islet tissue. Quart. J. Med., 6: 287-304, 1937.

94. Orci, L.: A portrait of the pancreatic beta cell.
     Diabetologia, 10: 163-187, 1974.

95. Orci, L., Amherdt, M., Henquin, J.C., Lambert, A.E., Unger,
     R.H. and Renold, A.E.: Pronase effect on pancreatic beta
     cell secretion and morphology. Science, 180: 647-649,
     1973.

96. Orci, L., Amherdt, M., Stauffacher, W., Like, A.A., Rouiller,
     C. and Renold, A.E.: Structural changes in membranes of
     beta cells exposed to alloxan and streptozotocin demon-
     strated by freeze-etching. Diabetes, 21 (Suppl. 1),
     326, 1972.

97. Orci, L., Like, A.A., Amherdt, M., Blondel, B., Kanazawa, Y.,
     Marliss, E.B., Lambert, A.E., Wollheim, C.B. and Renold, A.E.
     Monolayer cell culture of neonatal rat pancreas: an ultra-
     structural and biochemical study of functioning endocrine
     cells. J. Ultrastruct. Res., 43: 270-297, 1973.

98. Orci, L., Malaisse-Lagae, F., Ravazzola, M., Unger, R.H. and
     Renold, A.E.: The effect of exocrine pancreatic enzymes
     on islet cells junctions. Diabetes 23 (Suppl. 1), 339,
     1974.

99. Orci, L., Ravazzola, M., Amherdt, M. and Malaisse-Lagae, F.:
     The beta cell boundary. In Diabetes: International Diabetes
     Fed. VIII Congress, 1974.

100. Orci, L., Stauffacher, W., Dulin, W.E., Renold, A.E. and
      Rouiller, C.: Ultrastructural changes in alpha cells
      exposed to diabetic hyperglycemia. Observations made
      on pancreas of Chinese hamsters. Diabetologia, 6:
      199-206, 1970.

101. Orci, L., Stauffacher, W., Renold, A.E. and Rouiller, C.: In
      Current Topics on Glucagon. (M. Austoni, C. Scandellari, G.
      Federspil, and A. Trisotto, eds.) Padova, 15-30, 1971.

102. Orci, L., Unger, R. and Renold, A.E.: Structural basis for
      intercellular communications between cells of the islets
      of Langerhans. Experimentia 29: 777, 1973.

103. Orci, L., Unger, R.H. and Renold, A.E.: Structural coupling
      between pancreatic islet cells. Experientia (Basel),
      29: 1015-1018, 1973.

104. O'Sullivan, J.B. and Hurwitz, D.: Spontaneous remissions in
      early diabetes mellitus. Arch. Int. Med., 117: 769,
      1966.

105. O'Sullivan, J.B. and Mahan, C.M.: Prospective study of 352
      young patients with chemical diabetes. N. Eng. J. Med.,
      278: 1038, 1968.

106. Pavel, I.: Ereditatea in Diabet. Editura Academiei, Buchar-
      est, 1968.

107. Payton, B.W., Bennett, M.V.L. and Pappas, G.D.: Permeability
      and structure of junctional membranes at an electrotonic
      synapse. Science, 166: 1641-1643, 1969.

108. Pearse, J.: In Peptide Hormones. (J. Parsons, ed.) Plenum
      Press, in press.

109. Pinto da Silva, P. and Branton, D.: Membrane splitting in
      freeze-etching. J. Cell Biol. 45: 598-605, 1970.

110. Porte, D., Jr., Graber, A.L., Kuzuya, T. and William, R.H.:
      The effect of epinephrine on immunoreactive insulin levels
      in man. J. Clin. Invest. 45: 227-236, 1966.

111. Price, J.B., Takeshige, K., Max, M.H. and Voorhees, A.B.:
      Glucagon as the portal factor modifying hepatic regenera-
      tion. Surgery, 72: 74-82, 1972.

112. Reaven, G.M., Lerner, R.L., Stern, M.P. and Farquhar, J.:
      Role of insulin in endogenous hypertriglyceridemia. J.
      Clin. Invest. 46: 1756, 1967.

113. Renold, A.E., Cahill, G.C. and Gerritsen, G.C.: Second Brook
      Lodge Workshop on Spontaneous Diabetes in Laboratory Ani-
      mals. Diabetologia, 6: 153, 1970.

114. Renold, A.E. and Dulin, W.E.: Spontaneous diabetes in labora-
      tory animals. Diabetologia, 3: 63-64, 1967.

115. Renold, A.E., Rabinovitch, A., Wollheim, C.B., Kikuchi, M.,
      Gutzeit, A.H., Amherdt, M., Malaisse-Lagae, F. and Orci,
      L.: Spontaneous and experimental diabetic syndromes in
      animals. A re-evaluation of their usefulness for approach-
      ing the physiopathology of diabetes. In: Diabetes: Inter-
      national Diabetes Federation VIII Congress, 22-38, 1974.

116. Revel, J.P. and Karnovsky, M.J.: Hexagonal array of sub-units
      in intercellular junctions of the mouse heart and liver.
      J. Cell Biol. 33: C7-C12, 1967.

117. Robertson, R.P. and Porte, D.: The glucose receptor: A
      defective mechanism in diabetes mellitus distinct from the
      beta adrenergic receptor. J. Clin. Invest. 52: 870, 1973.

118. Rollo, J.: Cases of the Diabetes Mellitus. (2nd edition).
      London, 1798.

119. Roth, J.: Peptide hormone binding to receptors: A preview
      of direct studies in vitro. Metabolism, 22: 1059-1073,
      1973.

120. Ruche, W., Koerker, D.J. et al.: Proceedings of the symposium
      Advances in Human Growth Hormone Research. (S. Raiti, ed.)
      U.S.Government Printing Office, Baltimore, Maryland (in
      press).

121. Ryan, J.R., Balodimos, M.C., Chazan, B.I., Root, H.F., Marble,
      A., White, P. and Joslin, A.P. : Quarter century victory
      medal for diabetes: A follow-up of patients one to twenty
      years later. Metabolism, 19 (7): 493-501, 1970.

122. Scully, R. E. Case record of the Mass. General Hospital.
      New Eng. J. Med., 273: 41, 1965.

123. Samols, E., Tyler, J.M., and Marks, V.: In Glucagon (P.J.
      LeFebvre and R.H. Unger, eds.) Pergamon Press, 1972.

124. Singer, S.J., Nicolson, G.L.:   The fluid mosaic model of the
      structure of cell membranes.   Science, 175: 720-731, 1972.

125. Siperstein, M.D., Raskin, P. and Burns, H. :   Electron micro-
      scopic quantification of diabetic microangiopathy.
      Diabetes, 22 (7):514-524, 1973.

126. Siperstein, M.D., Unger, R.H., et al.:   Studies of muscle
      capillary basement membranes in normal subjects, diabetic
      and prediabetic patients.   J. Clin. Invest. 47: 1973, 1968.

127. Soskin, S., and Levine, R.:   Carbohydrate metabolism.   Univ.
      Chicago Press, 1946.

128. Spergel, G., Levy, L.J., et al.:   Glucose intolerance in the
      progeny of rats treated with single sub-diabetogenic dose
      of alloxan.   Metabolism, 20: 401, 1971.

129. Spiro, R.G.:   Glycoproteins: Their biochemistry, biology and
      role in human disease.   New Eng. J. Med.   281: 991-1001,
      1969.

130. Spiro, R.G. and Spiro, M.J.:   Effect of diabetes on the bio-
      synthesis of the renal glomerular basement membrane.
      Diabetes, 20: 641, 1971.

131. Stamler, J., Pick, R. and Katz, L.N.:   Experiences in assess-
      ing estrogen antiatherogenesis in the chick, the rabbit,
      and man.   Annals N.Y. Acad. Sci.   64: 596-619, 1956-57.

132. Steere, R.L.:   Electron microscopy of structural detail in
      frozen biological specimens.   J. Biophys. Biochem. Cytol.
      3: 45-60, 1957.

133. Steinberg, A.G.:   The genetics of diabetes: A review. Ann. N.Y.
      Acad. Sci. 82: 197-207, 1959.

134. Stout, R.W.:   Development of vascular lesions in insulin-treated
      animals fed a normal diet.   Brit. Med. J., 3: 685-687, 1970.

135. Tattersall, R.B.:   Mild diabetes with dominant inheritance.
      Quart. J. Med. 43: 339-357, 1974.

136. Tattersall, R.B. and Fajans, S.S.: A difference between the
      inheritance of classical juvenile onset and maturity-onset
      type diabetes of young people. Diabetes, 24: 44-53, 1975.

137. Trivelli, L.A., Ranney, H.M. and Lai, H.T.: Hemoglobin com-
     ponents in patients with diabetes mellitus. N. Eng. J. Med.
     284: 353-357, 1971.

138. University Group Diabetes Program: A study of the effects of
     hypoglycemic agents on vascular complications in patients
     with adult-onset diabetes. II. Mortality results. Diab-
     etes, 19 (Suppl. 1): 789-830, 1970.

139. Vail, W.J., Papahadjopoulos, D. and Moscarello, M.A.: Inter-
     action of a hydrophobic protein with liposomes evidence
     for particles seen in freeze-fracture as being proteins.
     Biophys. Biochim. Acta, 345: 463-467, 1974.

140. Vracko, R.: Basal lamina layering in diabetes mellitus. Evi-
     dence for accelerated rate of cell death and cell regener-
     ation. Diabetes, 24: 94, 1974.

141. Vracko, R., Benditt, E.P.: Capillary basal lamina thickening:
     Its relationship to endothelial cell death and replacement.
     J. Cell Biol., 47: 281-285, 1970.

142. Vracko, R. and Benditt, E.P.: Restricted replicative life
     span of diabetic fibroblasts in vitro: its relation to
     microangiopathy. Fed. Proc., 33: 607, 1974.

143. Vracko, R. and Benditt, E.P.: Manifestations of diabetes
     mellitus -- their possible relationships to an underlying
     cell defect. Am. J. Pathol., 75: 270, 1974.

144. Wellman, K.F., Bancato, P., et al.: Fine structure of pan-
     creatic islets of mice infected with the M-variant of the
     encephalomyocarditis virus. Diabetologia, 8: 349, 1972.

145. Whitfield, A.B.W., Crane, C.W., French, J.M. and Bayler, T.J.:
     Life without a pancreas. The Lancet, 675-677, 1965.

146. Williamson, J.R., Vogler, N.J. and Kilo, C.: Estimation of
     vascular basement membrane thickness. Diabetes, 18: 567,
     1967.

147. Willis, T.: Pharmaceutice Rationalis. Dring, Harper and
     Leight, London. 1679.